Management of the patient-ventilator system

A TEAM APPROACH

Management of the patient-ventilator system

A TEAM APPROACH

KATHREN V. MARTZ, B.S., R.N.

JERRY JOINER, B.S., R.R.T.

RODGER M. SHEPHERD, M.D., F.A.A.P.

ILLUSTRATED

The C. V. Mosby Company

ST. LOUIS • TORONTO • LONDON   1979

The C. V. Mosby Company
11830 Westline Industrial Drive, St. Louis, Missouri 63141

Library of Congress Cataloging in Publication Data

Martz, Kathren V   1938-
    Management of the patient-ventilator system.
    Bibliography: p.
    1. Respiratory insufficiency.   2.   Inhalation
therapy—Equipment and supplies.   3.   Inhalation
therapy.   I.   Joiner, Jerry, 1942-   joint author.
II.   Shepherd, Rodger M., joint author.   III.   Title.
IV.   Title: Patient-ventilator system.   [DNLM:
1. Respirators.   2. Respiration, Artificial.
WF26 M388m]
RC735.I5M37   615'.64   78-31819
ISBN 0-8016-3139-4

GW/CB/B 9 8 7 6 5 4   02/C/218

This book is dedicated to the physicians, nurses, and respiratory therapists in the small hospitals of northern California. We salute these colleagues and their marvelous devotion to patient care. We hope this book proves helpful to them in their care of ventilator patients.

It is also dedicated to three spouses and four offspring, who waited patiently as the authors struggled to get a preliminary version of this book into final form.

Preface

Offering yet another book on the management of the patient-ventilator system is a bit like selling sand at the seashore. In the past few years such texts and manuals have proliferated. Nevertheless, we believe that our offering meets a need not met before—the need to provide specific information required by a patient care team when faced with making decisions.

Knowledge of principles is essential in making correct decisions, but principles can be hard to remember in the heat of battle—or in the management of an acutely ill patient. This book serves as a quick reference and guide as well as a means of confirming the accuracy of one's decisions at these times.

The team concept is promoted throughout. Some areas of practice have traditionally "belonged" to nurses, others to physicians, still others to respiratory therapists. In the management of patients attached to ventilators, we believe that who makes a decision should be of less importance than making the correct decision—and doing so in a timely manner. Hence, to promote clarity of goals and the methods by which they will be achieved, we believe that the entire team should be involved in making decisions. Furthermore, we believe that the more information each discipline has about the ventilatory status of the patient, the better decisions made about other areas of patient care will be.

Unfortunately, the need to manage critically ill patients receiving ventilation will continue to grow. Therefore it seems reasonable to expect that all members of the patient care team need to have the information that we have attempted to provide.

The approach, the style, and the content of this book are the result of many years of clinical experience at the bedside, both managing and teaching the management of patient-ventilator systems. Obviously we have learned from many others in our professional careers, and if we do not seem to give them adequate credit, it is only because they have all done their jobs so well. The information presented here is the result of internalization of the learning and the experiences that we have shared with many others throughout the country.

This book was originally developed as part of a training project* de-

*An Educational Program for Treatment of Acute Respiratory Insufficiency, RFP NHLI-74-15, contract No. 1-HR-42964.

signed to reduce the incidence of severe respiratory failure in hospitalized adults. We are indebted to our contract officer, Dr. John Mathis, for the encouragement he gave us during that project.

In developing the book we often sought the advice of the following pulmonary specialists: Robert Fallat, M.D., Harvey Tucker, M.D., and Ronald Elkin, M.D. They offered many helpful suggestions. However, these experts must not be held accountable for positions we adapt that may be thought by some to be oversimplified or arbitrary.

Sandra Gordon, R.R.T., Gary Gregorcyk, R.R.T., Barbara Meyer, R.P.T., Mary Lou Vavra, R.N., and Sandra Crabtree, R.N., contributed to the first draft of the book and helped monitor its early use in field trials.

Kathren V. Martz
Jerry Joiner
Rodger M. Shepherd

Contents

x

How to use this book

Introduction The book is divided into two major sections—text (Parts One and Two) and exercises (Part Three).

The text The text consists of chapters that correspond to the various steps involved in attaching a patient to a ventilator and weaning him from one. Each of these steps and their sequence is shown in the chart on p. xv.

Within the text, some pages are distinctively marked. These pages provide a quick review of one of the phases of management of the patient-ventilator system and a procedure to follow. Decision making is facilitated by charts, tables, lists of equipment, and algorithms.

It is intended that these distinctively marked pages be revised periodically to meet local needs and to incorporate new and better techniques. Furthermore, practitioners may find it convenient to remove these perforated, punched pages for placement in a loose-leaf binder at the bedside.

The remainder of the pages in the text are intended for the clinician or student who is learning or reviewing the management of patients attached to ventilators. These pages provide background information not usually needed during actual patient care. However, we also discuss some preparations that should be considered in advance of actual patient care situations.

The exercises The exercises are learning experiences that can help clinicians use the text section of the book in actual patient care. Decisions are arbitrated by referring to the text. These exercises rely on simple simulation techniques and case discussions and can be used as models for review exercises ("fire drills") if the team has not had occasion to manage an actual ventilator patient for some time.

Each exercise provides learning goals and a lesson plan. Some of the exercises may be done without a resource person. Others are facilitated by having an instructor or resource person available. An "instructor" means anyone who is knowledgable in the area of ventilatory management and can be any member of the patient care team.

Exercise 1 is intended to serve as a pretest and as a post-test of the clinician's or student's knowledge of ventilatory parameters and mechanics. A student's copy and an instructor's copy are provided.

Exercise 2 is an exercise in the skills and equipment needed for the management of a patient requiring an artificial airway. An instructor is necessary.

Exercise 3 provides "self-guided tours" of various ventilators. These tours can be done without an instructor if the clinician or student is familiar with the basic principles of ventilator function. However, one instructor can facilitate the tours by supervising several individuals or teams simultaneously.

Exercise 4 is a series of "ventilator application situations" covering all the necessary steps in attaching a patient to, and weaning him from, a ventilator. An instructor is required for each of two or three teams.

Exercise 5 is directed more specifically at the process of weaning a patient from the ventilator.

Exercise 6 is an advanced ventilator exercise that allows the local expert to discuss areas not covered in the book or to make suggestions for modifications to meet local needs. Instructor and student versions are provided.

Organization of this book

The organization of this book is based on the following view of the sequence of tasks involved in mechanical ventilation of patients. The chapter number of each task is given in bold type.

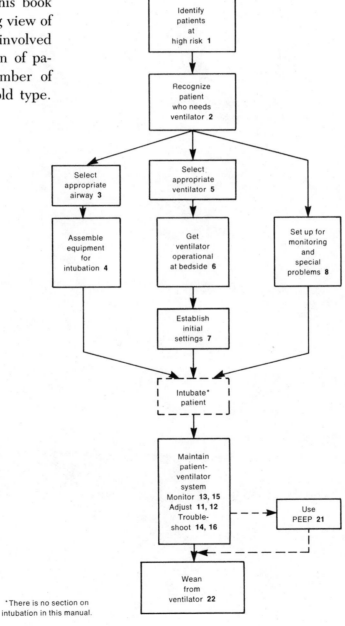

*There is no section on intubation in this manual.

PART ONE

Creating the patient-ventilator system

CHAPTER 1

Patients at special risk

Introduction The decision to intubate a patient and initiate mechanical ventilation should be made as *early* as possible. This means that patients at special risk of respiratory failure should be monitored for evidence of respiratory failure. What patients are at special risk? What should be monitored?

Patients at special risk One way to assess a patient's risk of respiratory failure is to ask yourself three questions about the patient:

Can he move air?
Can he move secretions?
Can he move blood?

Can he move air? Compare the patient's ability to breathe to your own. Does the patient have any problem that would make it harder to get air in and out of his lungs? Is the airway narrowed? Are the lungs diseased? Is the bellows mechanism (chest wall and diaphragm) intact? Are the muscles of respiration weak? Are those muscles being "driven" by the central nervous system (CNS), or is the patient obtunded?

Can he move secretions? Even if the patient can move air well enough to breathe, he may still have trouble moving secretions. Ask yourself if the patient can take a deep breath and expel it as rapidly as you can. Does it hurt to take a deep breath or cough? Are secretions too abundant or too thick for the patient to handle? Is the patient too obtunded to cough or protect himself against aspiration?

Can he move blood? Severe heart failure can cause pulmonary edema and respiratory distress. However, even milder degrees of heart failure or shock can mean that the patient has less energy to devote to moving air or clearing secretions. Shock can result in damage to the lungs. Low cardiac output aggravates the effect of "shunts" on arterial oxygen pressure (Pa_{O_2}). For these and other reasons, the patient whose blood cannot circulate is also at risk of respiratory failure.

Some examples The risk of respiratory failure is often underestimated in the following types of patients:

Obtunded or unconscious patients
Patients with thoracotomy or upper abdominal incisions

3

Patients with inhalation injuries (smoke, heat, chemicals, drowning)
Patients with acute respiratory infections superimposed on emphysema or chronic bronchitis
Patients with multiple trauma and shock
Patients with low cardiac output states
Additional risk exists if the patient is obese, smokes, or is in pain.

How to monitor? If you suspect that your patient may have trouble moving air, secretions, or blood, how do you monitor for early respiratory failure? In answering that question you should consider the definition of respiratory failure.

Definition Respiratory failure can be defined as (1) failure to keep arterial carbon dioxide pressure (Pa_{CO_2}) and pH within acceptable limits, (2) failure to keep Pa_{O_2} at an acceptable level, or (3) exhaustion of the patient while trying to maintain Pa_{CO_2} and Pa_{O_2} at tolerable levels.

High Pa_{CO_2} or low Pa_{O_2} usually occurs after the patient has exhausted himself trying to keep Pa_{O_2} and pH normal. This means that tests of respiratory effort, showing the degree of "fatigue" or "exhaustion," may provide the earliest evidence of respiratory failure.

Tests of "exhaustion" There are two measurements of the patient's respiratory reserve that can be determined through simple bedside tests: vital capacity (VC) and respiratory rate (f).

Vital capacity Vital capacity (VC), a very useful measure of ventilatory reserve, can be obtained with a simple mechanical spirometer or a calibrated bag.

A patient's normal VC usually falls in the range of 60 to 80 ml/kg of body weight. When VC falls below 20 ml/kg, sudden additional metabolic demands, such as those brought on by fever, restlessness, or anxiety, can trigger serious respiratory failure.

Vital capacity clinical guideline: VC = 60 to 80 ml/kg normally

If vital capacity is less than 20 ml/kg, be concerned and prepare to step up support.

A patient who cannot rapidly count aloud to 20 on exhalation after maximal inspiration has a greatly decreased vital capacity, and further evaluation should be made quickly.

Respiratory rate As the chest or the lungs become difficult to expand, the body attempts to compensate for the shallower breaths by increasing the number of breaths per minute. This happens very early in the respiratory disease. As a result, increased f can be an early clue to respiratory distress.

However, rapid respiration is fatiguing. Adults usually breathe with little effort at 10 to 15 breaths per minute. When the rate rises to 30, a large amount of energy is devoted to breathing. A sick person cannot sustain this rate indefinitely. When the patient is driven to breathe at a rate of 40, he will become exhausted very soon.

Respiratory rate clinical guideline: f = 10 to 15 for adults at rest

If greater than 25, be concerned and get other measurements.

If greater than 40, be concerned and prepare to ventilate.

Arterial blood gases   When the tests of "exhaustion" suggest respiratory failure, it is time to start checking arterial blood gases. They will serve to confirm the diagnosis of respiratory failure.

Pa_{O_2}   A Pa_{O_2} of 50 mm Hg, particularly if measured while the patient is breathing oxygen in concentrations greater than 40%, is reason for concern in some patients but not in others. Many patients with chronic lung disease have Pa_{O_2}s of about 40 mm Hg. Patients, however, who are "getting well" rather than "getting worse" may do nicely on a Pa_{O_2} of 50 mm Hg. Be cautious about relying on cyanosis as an indicator of Pa_{O_2}. Cyanosis is usually a very late sign of hypoxemia and may be misinterpreted because of poor lighting, anemia, or increased peripheral vascular resistance.

Pa_{O_2} clinical guideline: Pa_{O_2} is normally above 80 in a patient breathing room air.

If the Pa_{O_2} is 50 mm Hg or below in a patient receiving oxygen, be concerned and prepare to provide mechanical support.

Pa_{CO_2} and pH   A pH of less than 7.25 that is not caused by metabolic acidosis will be accompanied by a Pa_{CO_2} of 50 to 55. If the adequacy of ventilation cannot be reestablished immediately (for example, by reversal of narcotic effect or removal of mucus plugs) this level of pH can be life threatening. *Prepare to intubate* and ventilate mechanically. Since the signs of hypercarbia are common to many problems, they are unreliable for confirmation of acidosis. Acidosis should be suspected whenever arrhythmias, increased use of accessory muscles, diaphoresis, somnolence, or changes in heart rate and blood pressure exist in the presence of "mild respiratory distress." Confirmation by blood gas determination is essential.

Pa_{CO_2} and pH clinical guidelines: Pa_{CO_2} is normally 40 ± 3; pH is normally 7.40 ± 0.03

When Pa_{CO_2} rises above 50 and pH falls below 7.25, the patient probably will need help in ventilating.

Trends are the best evidence   Sometimes we are forced to evaluate a patient quickly and decide about mechanical ventilation based on his condition at one point in time. In such a situation we must use guidelines based on experience.

However, it is usually possible to make better decisions when we have access to serial observations. Serial observations permit us to compare the patient with himself. For example, a patient with chronic obstructive pulmonary disease (COPD) may have a Pa_{CO_2} of 50 and Pa_{O_2} of 50. Serial observations may show that he is adjusted to these values and that they remain constant day in and day out.

On the other hand, as an asthmatic patient becomes exhausted, his Pa_{CO_2} may change from 35 to 45 within an hour.

When in doubt, monitor   If recognizing trends makes for better decisions, then better decisions depend on early monitoring. Monitoring early usually means monitoring as soon as you are aware that the patient is at special risk. Recognizing that the patient is at special risk means knowing the special-risk patient groups and asking yourself:

Can he move air?

Can he move secretions?

Can he move blood?

CHAPTER 2

Indications for mechanical ventilation

Introduction A patient being ventilated is a major responsibility for the health care team. There may be understandable reluctance to attach a patient to a ventilator and assume the responsibility of management. However, the experienced team realizes that "earlier is better."

The need for ventilation of the apneic patient is obvious and requires no discussion. Instead, this section will consider the use of mechanical ventilation of the patient with increasing respiratory failure.

Indications In most situations, mechanical ventilation should be considered when:

Pa_{O_2} cannot be maintained above 50 mm Hg by increasing the fractional concentration of inspired oxygen ($F_{I_{O_2}}$)

Pa_{CO_2} rises above 50 and causes the pH to drop below 7.25

Ventilation becomes inefficient and exhausting (respiratory rate over 30 or vital capacity less than 20 ml/kg)

Special cases There are a few special cases in which these rules might be interpreted in light of the situation. For example:

Patients with COPD may have become well adjusted to a Pa_{O_2} below 50 mm Hg. Use other indications for intubating and ventilating such patients.

Patients with drug overdose can be very deceiving. The patient's condition can suddenly get worse if more drug is absorbed from the intestine. If the patient appears obtunded, intubation and ventilation may be indicated as a precaution—even before the criteria listed above are satisfied.

Neuromuscular diseases (for example myasthenia gravis or Guillain-Barré syndrome) may progress in a way that allows you to predict that the respiratory rate will soon exceed 30 or the VC will drop below 20 ml/kg. When the trend of serial observations points in this direction, intubation and mechanical ventilation are indicated.

Patients with flail chest will usually require controlled ventilation if any of the following apply:

Large flail segment (for example, over 5 cm in diameter)

Pre-existing lung disease
Lung contusion on x-ray film
Compromised cough
Multiple injuries

CHAPTER 3

Selection of airway

Introduction   Mechanical ventilation requires an air-tight connection between the ventilator and the trachea. An orotracheal tube, nasotracheal tube, or tracheostomy tube can be used for this purpose. Each kind of tube has certain advantages. However, low cuff pressure is the most important consideration.

Cuff compliance   The overriding consideration in the choice of an airway is the compliance of the cuff. The cuff should be large enough and soft enough to control leaks with cuff inflation pressures less than 25 mm Hg.

Periodic deflation has been advocated by some to reduce cuff injury to the trachea. However, there is no evidence yet that tracheal blood flow is improved by this maneuver. Furthermore, the maneuver is time consuming, the large leak created results in less effective ventilation of the patient, and the patient is at risk of aspiration while the cuff is deflated.

The tube itself   The tube should be made of a nonreactive polymer; an ideal material would be soft and flexible and mold easily to the contours of the airway. Such molding reduces the tendency of the tube to exert sharp destructive pressure on certain points in the pharynx and larynx. The tube should have a radiopaque marker that defines the tip.

Types of tubes   The three types of tubes in common use are:
1. *Orotracheal tube*. This tube usually is used for emergencies; it may be left in 12 to 18 hours. After reevaluation it may be left in longer, but it is the least comfortable tube for the patient. It induces salivation, making oral care difficult.
2. *Nasotracheal tube*. This tube is much preferred for comfort, although its diameter may have to be smaller because of some patients' narrow posterior nares. Nasotracheal tubes may be left in place for days to weeks, although any single tube should probably be changed periodically.
3. *Tracheostomy tube*. Tracheal toilet is easiest when this tube is used, and comfort is most enhanced. The area around the stoma requires frequent cleaning, occasionally (every 4 to 8 hours) with a mild (¼%) acetic acid solution.

CHAPTER 4

Preparing for intubation

Introduction   Whether the intubation is elective or emergent, having the appropriate equipment assembled should facilitate the procedure. We suggest that you have the equipment assembled on a tray or drawer of a cart for easy access. Furthermore, we recommend that this equipment be checked on a routine basis along with other emergency equipment.

Other considerations   Obviously, once the patient is intubated, the ventilator should be ready for use. Please consult the flow sheet for other steps that should be taken at this time.

Sample list of equipment needed for intubation

1. Cardiac monitor
2. Oxygen source
3. Oxygen face mask
4. Resuscitation bag and mask
5. Suction source, catheters, and tonsil tip sucker
6. Sedatives and muscle relaxants
7. Anesthetic spray
8. Sterile gloves
9. McGill forceps
10. Oropharyngeal bite block or airway
11. Nasogastric tube and catheter tip syringe
12. Stylette
13. Tube stabilization equipment
14. Laryngoscope with curved and straight blades
15. Endotracheal tubes
16. Sterile, water-soluble lubricant
17. Syringe for cuff inflation
18. Rubber-tipped clamp
19. Connectors

We suggest that you modify this list to suit the needs of your institution.

Equipment needed for intubation

Cardiac monitor   Intubation may intensify existing arrhythmias or produce new ones. All patients are subject to these arrhythmias and should be monitored.

Oxygen source   A reliable source of oxygen at 50 pounds/square inch (PSI) is required. Two outlets should be available, since one is needed for attaching the ventilator and another for connecting the manual resuscitation bag.

Compressed air   Some ventilators require a source of compressed gas for delivery of the minute ventilation. If your ventilator is one of them, then compressed air at 50 PSI should also be available.

Resuscitation bag and mask   The patient should be well oxygenated immediately prior to intubation. Oxygen consumption is increased because of an anxiety-induced sympathetic response. The patient's airway and ventilatory ability are impaired during intubation. Therefore, preoxygenation and repeated reoxygenation every few minutes are essential during intubation. A skilled practitioner can ventilate a patient quite effectively with a mask and bag.

Suction source, catheters, and tonsil tip sucker   Intubation may induce vomiting; therefore, be prepared to reposition the patient quickly and to clear the vomitus from the airway to prevent aspiration. The suction catheter selected for use should be approximately half the diameter of the endotracheal tube.

Anesthetic spray   Densensitization of the pharynx will decrease patient discomfort and may allow an easier intubation.

Sterile gloves   Although the upper airway is not sterile, we recommend that sterile gloves be used during intubation. Airway infections are not uncommon, and every possible precaution should be taken.

McGill forceps   Nasotracheal intubation may be facilitated by the use of forceps sufficiently long to reach the tube as it passes down the posterior pharynx.

Oropharyngeal bite block or airway   Many patients will reflexly bite down on the tube after placement. An oral bite block should be taped in place until the patient is fully alert and cooperative.

Nasogastric tube, catheter tip, and syringe   If the stomach is not decompressed prior to intubation, the risk of aspiration is increased. Whether continued nasogastric decompression is needed should be determined after the patient's condition is stabilized. Patients using great inspiratory effort open the esophagus because of increased negative intrathoracic pressure, and gastric dilatation can occur.

Stylette   Endotracheal tubes may need "shaping" with a stylette for placement. The stylette should have a nontraumatic distal end to prevent tracheal trauma.

Tube stabilization equipment   Once in place, the tube must be securely stabilized to prevent displacement as well as oropharyngeal tracheal damage. Benzoin may be useful in providing better tape adhesion. If the tube is connected to a ventilator, the ventilator tubing must be supported to prevent tugging on the airway.

Laryngoscope, curved and straight blades

Intubators have personal preferences as to type of blade used. Straight and curved should be available. Batteries and bulbs providing the light source should be routinely checked, and an extra supply should be immediately available.

Endotracheal tubes

Two sterile tubes of the desired size with intact cuffs should be immediately available. One should be kept at the bedside for emergency reintubation.

Sterile water, soluble lubricant

Coating the endotracheal tube with a lubricant should make passage of the tube easier. Some intubators prefer to use an anesthetic lubricant such as lidocaine (Xylocaine) ointment.

Syringe for cuff inflation

A syringe of appropriate size should be kept at the bedside of each patient intubated.

Rubber-tipped clamp

Although most cuffed tubes have an attached seal for the inflatable cuff, on occasion this seal may malfunction. A nontraumatic clamp may be useful in that situation.

Connectors

Specific types and sizes of connectors depend on the endotracheal tube that is used. All should be of an appropriate size and diameter to connect the tube either to a resuscitation bag or to the ventilator tubing.

Stethoscope

Immediately after intubation, auscultation of the chest should be done to verify inflation of both lungs.

CHAPTER 5

Guide to selection of ventilators

Introduction Two types of ventilators are in general use today: pressure-cycled and volume-cycled. Most hospitals have both types available. Most patients who require continuous ventilation can be managed successfully with either a pressure-cycled or a volume-cycled ventilator. However, each type has some advantages over the other, and each ventilator has its own unique characteristics.

Guidelines The following algorithm is one way to consider selection of the most desirable ventilator.

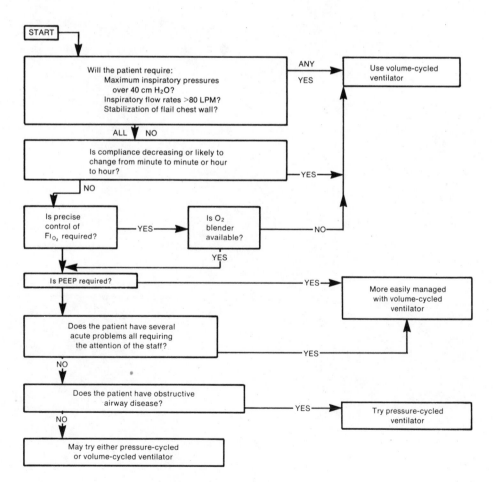

Comments on the guide to selection of ventilators

> Will the patient require:
> Maximum inspiratory pressures
> over 40 cm H_2O?
> Inspiratory flow rates >80 LPM?
> Stabilization of flail chest wall?

Although newer models of pressure ventilators can deliver flow rates and create pressures similar to the capabilities of volume ventilators, many pressure ventilators cannot.

If a maximum inspiratory pressure (MIP) greater than 40 cm H_2O is required to deliver an adequate tidal volume, older pressure ventilators may be incapable of meeting the need.

Patients with severe bronchospasm (status asthmaticus) or "stiff lungs" (for example, shock lung) often require inflation pressures above 40 cm H_2O.

Flow rates are also limited on older models of pressure ventilators. Therefore, patients with stiff lungs requiring high pressures with fairly rapid inflation may need faster flow rates than are possible with a pressure ventilator.

Also, large patients (heavier than 100 kg) may require inspiratory flow rates (IFR) greater than 80 liters per minute (LPM).

If the patient's spontaneous minute volume ($V_T \times f$) exceeds 30 to 40 LPM, his IFR is probably in excess of 80 LPM.

Stabilization of a flail segment of chest wall is more easily accomplished with a volume ventilator. A volume ventilator also does a better job of expanding the underlying contused lung. Guaranteed volume permits more precise control of Pa_{CO_2}. With large, satisfying tidal volumes and a low Pa_{CO_2}, the patient is not inclined to breathe spontaneously and produce destabilizing paradoxical movements of the flail segment.

> Is compliance decreasing or likely to
> change from minute to minute or hour
> to hour?

As secretions accumulate and atelectasis occurs, compliance decreases. Other lung diseases such as pulmonary edema and shock lung can also cause decreased compliance. If a patient with decreasing compliance is being ventilated with a pressure-cycled ventilator, the V_T decreases unless the inflation pressure is increased. If the V_T decreases, both ventilation and oxygenation may suffer. Obviously, control of the V_T is easier when a volume ventilator is used.

Is precise control of $F_{I_{O_2}}$ required?		Is O_2 blender available?

Precise $F_{I_{O_2}}$ control on many pressure ventilators is not possible without an oxygen blender. Oxygen delivery from a 50 PSI source directly to a pressure ventilator may result in a delivered oxygen concentration of 40% to 90% in the air-mix mode. Precise control of $F_{I_{O_2}}$ with pressure-cycled ventilators requires the use of an oxygen blender.

Is PEEP required?

Positive end-expiratory pressure (PEEP) is more easily managed on a volume ventilator. In addition, patients requiring PEEP generally have complex, multi-system organic problems making general management simpler when a volume-cycled ventilator is used.

Does the patient have several acute problems all requiring the attention of the staff?

If the patient is acutely ill with multiple problems each requiring considerable attention, it will be easier to manage the patient by using a volume ventilator. It will also be safer.

Alarms are available to warn the busy staff about changes in machine function and patient response. Delivery of the desired volume continues despite changes in lung compliance.

Does the patient have obstructive airway disease?

Tapered inspiratory flow tends to ventilate obstructed airways better. Thus pressure ventilators may provide better ventilation for these patients. Many of them have pressure-cycled ventilators at home and are more familiar with, and thus less anxious about, their use. In addition, previous hospitalizations have probably acquainted these patients with pressure-cycled ventilators for delivery of aerosol medication, intermittent positive pressure breathing (IPPB) treatments, or continuous ventilation.

Table 1 Comparison of representative pressure-cycled and volume-cycled ventilators

Parameters	Pressure-cycled (Bird Mark 7)	Volume-cycled (Bennett MA-1)
Approximate cost	Ventilator $900 Spirometer 300 Blender 350 PEEP 75 Cascade 250	Complete $6400
Pressure	0-40 cm H_2O Preset, constant; determines depth of inspiration	0-80 cm H_2O Resultant, therefore variable; compensates for compliance and resistance changes
Volume	Resultant, therefore variable; changes as compliance or resistance changes	Preset, constant; determines depth of inspiration
Flow rate	Uncalibrated, limited to 80 LPM; decreases greatly with increasing pressure	Calibrated 10-100 LPM Peak flow decreases only slightly with increasing pressure
Oxygen concentration ($F_{I_{O_2}}$)	100%, or air mix—60%-80%; O_2 blender may be used for 21%-100%	21%-100% Dial adjustment
Respiration rate	Set with apnea control (*expiration time*)	1 breath/3 min to 60/min Dial adjustment
Sensitivity	Adjustable from self-cycle to approximately −10 cm H_2O	Adjustable from self-cycle to −10 cm H_2O Indicator light
Sigh	Manual; push in manual timing rod and hold until desired pressure is given	Programmed volume, frequency, and multiple Sigh indicator light and pressure limit
PEEP	May be added but cumbersome and difficult to regulate; not recommended	0-15 cm H_2O Uncalibrated dial adjustment
Humidifier	500 ml Micronebulizer with wrap-around, fixed temperature; heater may be added or Bennett Cascade may be used	Cascade I: bubble-through, blow over humidifier with variable temperature Cascade II: servo-controlled humidifier with patient airway gas temperature control and display
Spirometer	Draeger or Bennett Spirometer may be added or Wright may be used	Bennett bellows type 0-2200 ml, 200 ml increments Low volume and rate alarm

Table 2 Comparison of two pressure-cycled ventilators

Parameters	Bennett	Bird	Function
Pressure	All models	All models	Sets inspiratory pressure limit
Inspiratory flow	Preset according to pressure setting	All models	Flow rate and inspiratory time
Peak flow	PR II: adjustable from 15-100 LPM	None	Limits peak inspiratory flow rate
Sensitivity	PR I, PR II	All models	Adjusts response of machine to inspiratory effort
Air dilution	PR I, PR II*	Mark 7, 8, 9, 14	100% O_2 or 60%* O_2
Nebulization			Adjusts rate of nebulization during:
Inspiratory	PR II	Not adjustable	Inspiration
Expiratory	PR II	None	Expiration
Constant	PR I, PV-3P, AP-4	None	Continuous
Terminal flow	PR II	Mark 10, 14	Compensates for leaks
Negative pressure†	PR I-A, PR II	Mark 8	Exerts negative pressure on exhalation
Rate (apnea)	PR I, PR II	Mark 7, 8, 9, 10, 14	Sets controlled respiratory rate; I : E ratio 1 : 1.5 for Bennett, variable for Bird
Expiratory time	PR II	See rate	Prolongs exhalation time and alters I : E ratio

*In "air dilute" position, the Bird models may actually deliver 50% to 80% oxygen, depending on the other settings. Bennett models may deliver 60% to 80% in the "air mix" mode.

† Negative pressure—not recommended because of tendency to promote alveolar collapse and atelectasis.

Table 3 Comparisons of volume ventilators according to functional characteristics

Characteristic	Bennett MA-1	Ohio 560	Searle VVA
Adjustable parameters (preset)			
Tidal volume	100-2200 ml	100-2200 ml	300-2200 ml
Respiratory rate	6-60/min unmodified; 1 breath/3 min to 60/min if modified for IMV	See "Expiratory time" and "Inspiratory flow rate"	5-60/min; IDV unit: 1 per 2 breaths to 1 per 100 breaths
Inspiratory flow rate			
at 0 cm H_2O	15-100 LPM	10-250 LPM	20-200 LPM
at 40 cm H_2O	75 LPM	100 LPM	20-200 LPM
Expiratory time	—	0.5 to 7 sec	—
O_2 concentration	21%-100%	21%-100%	21%-100%
PEEP	0-15 cm H_2O	0-10 cm H_2O	0-20 cm H_2O
Inflation hold	—	0-2 sec	0-3 sec
Sensitivity	−0.1 to −10 cm H_2O; manually PEEP compensated	−0.2 to −10 cm H_2O and off	−0.2 to −20 cm H_2O and off; PEEP compensated
Expiratory retard	Yes	No	No
Sigh volume	100-2200 ml	0-4000 ml	0-2200 ml
Sigh frequency	4-15 per hour	1 every 2-10 min	1 every 1-10 min
Sigh multiple	1, 2, or 3	—	1, 2, or 3
Alarms			
O_2 supply	Audible and visible	Visible (reservoir—not line pressure)	Audible and visible
Airway disconnect			
Low pressure	—	Audible and visible	Audible and visible
Low volume	Audible (top of spirometer)	—	Spirometer
Failure to cycle	—	Audible and visible (fail-safe valve opens)	Audible and visible
Power disconnect	Audible (spirometer)	Audible	Audible and visible
High pressure	Audible and visible	Audible and visible	Audible and visible
Pressure relief	Valve without separate alarm	Valve without separate alarm and valve with alarm, audible and visible	Valve with separate alarm, audible and visible
I:E ratio	Visible	—	Visual short exhalation
End-expiratory pressure	—	—	Visual (except PEEP preset)
Indicators			
Assist	Light	Light	Light (PEEP compensated)
Sigh	Light	Bellow (visible)	—
Respiratory rate	—	Meter	Digital
I:E ratio	—	—	Digital

CHAPTER 6

Ventilator readiness

Introduction When the decision has been made to intubate a patient and initiate mechanical ventilation, the nurse and the respiratory therapist should make certain preparations. They should work from checklists to avoid duplication of effort and yet assure that all the necessary preparations are made.

Assumptions The following plan is based on four assumptions:
1. Continuous ventilation has been ordered by the physician.
2. The type of ventilator has been specified.
3. The patient has been or will be intubated shortly.
4. Both respiratory therapist and nurse are available to assemble and check out equipment.

Tasks for the nurse We suggest that the nurse assure that the following are available at the bedside:
1. ECG monitor
2. Suction source, catheters, gloves, and tonsil tip sucker
3. Syringe appropriate for cuff size
4. Rubber-tipped clamp
5. Stethoscope
6. Magic slate or other means of communication for the patient.
7. Arterial blood gas (ABG) determination capability
8. Intubation tray
9. Distilled sterile water
10. Tracheostomy tray*
11. Chest tube insertion tray*

Tasks for the therapist The therapist should concentrate first on assembling all the equipment that may be stored under his or her supervision. When all the equipment has been brought to the bedside, the therapist should assemble the equipment and make sure it functions properly.

*These items need not be at the bedside, but should be immediately available in the intensive care unit (ICU).

Equipment list

1. Oxygen source
2. Ventilator
3. Spirometer (Wright, Draeger, Bennett)
4. Humidifier (Cascade, Searle, Ohio, USN)
5. Oxygen analyzer
6. Rubber test lung
7. Oxygen blender (if pressure-cycled ventilator)
8. Distilled sterile water
9. Resuscitation bag
10. Two endotracheal tubes (size appropriate for patient)
11. Connectors, adapters, and dead-space tubing

Check out procedure

Keep the following points in mind when you check out a ventilator for readiness:

1. Ventilator correctly assembled
2. Humidifier filled, heater plugged in, and thermostat set
3. Power disconnect alarm functional
4. Proper electrical connection made
5. Low pressure alarm functional
6. Oxygen hose connectd to 50 PSI source
7. Oxygen concentration accurate
8. Failure-to-cycle alarm functional
9. High pressure alarm and relief valve functional
10. I : E ratio alarm and indicator functional
11. Leaks absent in:
    a. Humidifier
    b. Tubing connections
    c. Tubing
    d. Exhalation diaphragm
    e. Manifold
    f. Nebulizer
    g. Test lung
12. Sigh volume, frequency, and multiple selector functional
13. Gas temperature appropriate
14. Accessories available

The following sections outline procedures for performance testing specific ventilators.

Bennett MA-1

Introduction   The following procedure assumes that a Bennett MA-1 volume ventilator has been assembled correctly and that all necessary accessories have been attached to support a patient being mechanically ventilated.

Equipment needed
1. Rubber test lung
2. Spirometer (Wright, Draeger)
3. Oxygen analyzer

Steps
1. Fill the cascade humidifier with sterile distilled water.
   Turn the thermostat to a setting of 5.
   Plug the power cord into a 110-volt AC outlet.
   Check the inside front panel of the ventilator to verify that audible pressure alarm switch is turned on.
   Turn spirometer alarm on, with metering stick at 500 ml.
2. Adjust ventilator controls as follows:

$$F_{I_{O_2}} = 0.6$$
$$\text{Tidal volume} = 600 \text{ ml}$$
$$\text{Respiratory rate} = 10 \text{ BPM}$$
$$\text{Inspiratory flow rate} = 25 \text{ LPM}$$
$$\text{Inspiratory pressure limit} = 80 \text{ cm } H_2O$$
$$\text{All other settings} = \text{off}$$
$$\text{Power switch} = \text{on}$$

   ☐ The audible and visual alarm should activate, indicating that the high pressure oxygen hose has not been attached to an oxygen source.
3. Attach the high pressure oxygen hose to a 50 PSI oxygen source.
   ☐ The audible and visual alarms should turn off.
   ☐ The green oxygen light should activate.
   ☐ The spirometer alarm should sound 1 minute from the time it is turned on, indicating that the test lung is not attached.
4. Attach an O_2 analyzer to the Y piece of the patient circuit. Attach a rubber test lung to the analyzer sampling T.
   ☐ The spirometer alarm should stop when the next breath is exhaled.
5. Depress each of the indicator lights at the top of the instrument panel.
   ☐ Each light should turn on if the bulb is functional.
6. Allow the test lung to be ventilated for 2 minutes.
   Check the oxygen analyzer reading.
   ☐ The reading should agree ±5% with the oxygen setting on the ventilator. (If it does not, calibrate the analyzer for accuracy at 30% and 100%. Check linearity at 60%. Repeat step 6.)
7. Manually compress the test lung and hold for 30 seconds.
   ☐ The audible and visual high pressure alarms should activate with each inspiratory cycle. (If 80 cm H_2O is not reached, check for leaks and repeat.)

☐ The spirometer alarm should sound in approximately 20 seconds after the first cycle that delivers less than 500 ml.

☐ Check the spirometer for delivered volume. An internal safety mechanism should prevent the entire preset tidal volume from being delivered.

8. Adjust ventilator controls as follows:

Respiratory rate = 60
    Peak flow = minimum

☐ The I:E ratio alarm should activate with each machine cycle.

9. Adjust ventilator controls as follows:

Respiratory rate = minimum
    Peak flow = 25 LPM
        Sensitivity = turn clockwise until machine self-cycles; then turn counter-clockwise until self-cycling stops, and continue for one-half turn

Manually compress the test lung and release abruptly.

☐ The needle of the inspiratory pressure gauge should deflect to approximately -2 cm H_2O.

☐ The ventilator should cycle to inspiration and the orange assist light should activate.

10. Check the tidal volume as indicated on the spirometer.

☐ The tidal volume should be approximately equal to the tidal volume setting of the ventilator.

Comment: If the tidal volume does not correspond, suspect a leak or a malfunctioning spirometer. Double-check with another spirometer.

11. Check the temperature gauge.

☐ The temperature should be approximately body temperature 15 to 20 minutes after the thermostat is turned on.

☐ Adjust the setting as appropriate.

12. Prepare the ventilator for connection to the patient.

☐ Adjust all ventilator settings according to the guidelines provided.

Searle VVA

Introduction   The following procedure assumes that a Searle VVA volume ventilator has been assembled correctly and that all necessary accessories have been attached to support a patient being mechanically ventilated. (This procedure does not include the use of the ventilation mode controller or battery pack.)

Equipment needed
1. Rubber test lung
2. Spirometer (Wright, Draeger)
3. Oxygen analyzer

Steps
1. Fill the humidifier with sterile distilled water.
   Turn the thermostat to mid-range.
   Plug the heater into the power source on the back of the ventilator.
2. Adjust ventilator controls as follows:

$$F_{I_{O_2}} = 0.3$$
$$\text{Respiratory rate} = 10$$
$$\text{Tidal volume} = 500 \text{ ml}$$
$$\text{Inspiratory flow rate} = 20 \text{ LPM}$$
$$\text{Inspiratory pressure alarm} = 50 \text{ cm } H_2O$$
$$\text{Inspiratory pressure relief} = 100 \text{ cm } H_2O$$
$$\text{All other settings} = \text{off}$$
$$\text{Power switch} = \text{on}$$

   ☐ The audible and visual power disconnect alarm should activate, indicating that the power cord has not been plugged in.
3. Plug power cord into 110 volt AC outlet.
   ☐ The power disconnect alarm should turn off.
   ☐ The ventilator should begin cycling.
   ☐ The fan alarm should stop after a few machine cycles. (If it continues, check the fan filter for clogging.)
   ☐ The low-inspiratory-pressure alarm will activate, indicating that the test lung is not attached.
   ☐ The low-oxygen-pressure alarm will activate, indicating that the high-pressure oxygen hose has not been attached to an oxygen source.
4. Attach the high-pressure oxygen hose to a 50 PSI oxygen source.
   ☐ The oxygen alarm should turn off.
5. Attach an O_2 analyzer to the Y piece of the patient circuit.
   Attach a rubber test lung to the analyzer sampling T.
   ☐ The low-inspiratory-pressure alarm will turn off.
6. Allow the test lung to be ventilated for 2 minutes.
   Check the oxygen analyzer reading.
   ☐ The reading should agree ±5% with the oxygen setting on the ventilator. (If it does not, calibrate the analyzer for accuracy at 30% and 100%. Check linearity at 60%. Repeat step 6.)
7. Set the spirometer warning level to 400 ml.

The spirometer should now begin recording each exhaled volume.

☐ The tidal volume recorded should be approximately equal to the tidal volume setting of the ventilator.

8. Check the I:E ratio display.

☐ The I:E ratio that is desired is 1:2. Adjust the inspiratory flow rate until this ratio is achieved.

9. Depress the button labelled "Press to test."

☐ All of the indicator lights will light if the bulbs are functional.

10. Disconnect the inspiratory tubing from the patient side of the manifold outlet manually for 20 seconds.

☐ The audible and visual failure-to-cycle alarm should activate after 15 seconds.

Reconnect the inspiratory tubing and reset the alarm.

11. Adjust the ventilator controls as follows:

Respiratory rate = 30
Inspiratory flow rate = minimum

☐ The short exhalation light should activate with each cycle.

☐ The I:E ratio should now read less than 1:1

12. Adjust ventilator controls as follows:

Respiratory rate = 10
Inspiratory flow rate = adequate to achieve an I:E ratio of 1:2

13. Restrict the test lung to create inflation pressures of 50 cm H_2O.

☐ The audible and visual high-inspiratory-pressure alarm should activate as the pressure exceeds 50 cm H_2O during each inspiratory cycle.

14. Remove the test lung.

Occlude the outlet of the patient circuit.

☐ The audible and visual inspiratory-pressure-relief alarm should activate with each cycle.

☐ The inspiratory pressure should reach 100 cm H_2O during each in-inspiratory cycle. (If it does not, check for leaks.)

15. Occlude the tubing beyond the exhalation valve near the end of the exhalation phase. This will maintain some positive pressure in the circuit. Release this occlusion during the inspiratory phase.

☐ The end-expiratory pressure alarm should activate, indicating that a level of PEEP exists even though no PEEP is set by the ventilator control. (This may be caused by water collecting in the expiratory tubing or by kinking of the expiratory tubing.)

16. Turn the patient-triggering-effort dial to minimum. Manually compress the test lung and release abruptly.

☐ The needle of the pressure gauge should deflect to -0.5 to -2 cm H_2O before the ventilator cycles to inspiration.

☐ The amber assist light should activate, indicating a patient-assisted breath.

17. Check the temperature gauge.
    □ The temperature should be approximately at body temperature 15 to 20 minutes after the thermostat has been turned on.
18. Prepare the ventilator for connection to the patient.
    □ Adjust all ventilator settings according to guidelines provided.

Ohio 560

Introduction The following procedure assumes that an Ohio 560 volume ventilator has been assembled correctly and that all necessary accessories have been attached to support a patient being mechanically ventilated.

Equipment needed
1. Rubber test lung
2. Spirometer (Wright, Draeger)
3. Oxygen analyzer

Steps
1. Fill the humidifier with sterile distilled water.
   Turn the thermostat to a setting of 5.
   Plug the heater into a 110-volt AC outlet.
2. Adjust ventilator controls as follows:

   $$F_{I_{O_2}} = 0.3$$
   Tidal volume $= 500$ ml
   Inspiratory flow $= 2$
   Expiratory time $= 3$ seconds
   High pressure alarm $= 50$ cm H_2O
   Pressure relief $=$ closed
   Patient effort $=$ maximum
   Power switch $=$ on

3. Plug the ventilator power cord into a 110-volt AC outlet.
   ☐ The ventilator should begin cycling.
   ☐ The audible and visual oxygen alarms should activate, indicating that the high pressure oxygen hose has not been attached to an oxygen source.
   ☐ The low-pressure visual and audible alarms should activate, indicating that the test lung has not been attached.
4. Attach the high-pressure oxygen hose to a 50 PSI oxygen source.
   ☐ The oxygen alarm should turn off.
5. Attach an oxygen analyzer to the Y piece of the patient circuit. Attach a rubber test lung to the analyzer sampling T.
   ☐ The low-pressure alarm should turn off.
6. Allow the test lung to be ventilated for 2 minutes.
   Check the oxygen analyzer reading.
   ☐ The reading should agree ±5% with the oxygen setting on the ventilator. (If it does not, calibrate the analyzer for accuracy at 30% and 100%. Check linearity at 60%. Repeat step 6.)
7. Push and hold in the manual exhalation button while occluding the patient outlet manually.
   ☐ Fail-to-cycle alarm (audible and visual) should activate in approximately 15 seconds.
   Release patient outlet and reconnect test lung.
8. Push in and hold the manual inhalation button.
   ☐ The pressure relief valve should *not* be leaking.

Comment: If the pressure does not reach 100 cm H_2O, a leak is present in the circuit.

☐ Fail-to-cycle alarm should activate in approximately 8 seconds.

9. Push in and hold the manual inhalation button again.

☐ The high-pressure alarm (audible and visual) should activate as the pressure exceeds 50 cm H_2O.

10. Adjust the ventilator controls as follows:

$F_{I_{O_2}} = 0.6$
Pressure relief = 60 cm H_2O

11. Manually compress the test lung until an inspiratory cycle creates at least 60 cm H_2O pressure, and hold it through two inspiratory cycles.

☐ The pressure relief valve should operate when 60 cm H_2O is reached. It should be heard leaking.

☐ The high-pressure alarm should activate as 50 cm H_2O is reached during the second inspiratory cycle.

☐ Check the oxygen analyzer. The reading should agree ±5% of the oxygen setting on the ventilator.

12. Increase the expiratory time to 7 seconds. Adjust the patient-triggering-effort dial to 2. Manually compress the test lung. Wait for the pressure gauge needle to drop to zero. Then release the test lung abruptly.

☐ As the lung is released, the needle of the pressure gauge should travel to approximately −2 cm H_2O.

☐ The machine should cycle to inspiration.

☐ The patient-trigger light should activate.

Comment: If this does not occur, set the patient-triggering-effort dial at 1 and repeat.

13. Check the tidal volume as indicated on the spirometer.

☐ The tidal volume should be approximately equal to the tidal volume setting of the ventilator.

Comment: If the tidal volume does not correspond, suspect a leak or a malfunctioning spirometer. Double-check with another spirometer.

14. Check temperature gauge.

☐ The temperature should be approximately body temperature 15 to 20 minutes after the thermostat has been turned on. Adjust setting as appropriate.

15. Prepare the ventilator for connection to the patient.

☐ Adjust all ventilator settings according to the guidelines provided.

Bird Mark VII

Introduction   The following procedure assumes that a Bird Mark VII pressure-cycled ventilator has been correctly assembled and that all necessary accessories have been attached to support a patient being mechanically ventilated.

Equipment needed
1. Rubber test lung
2. Spirometer (Wright, Draeger)
3. Oxygen analyzer
4. Chronometer

Steps
1. Fill the humidifier with sterile distilled water.
   Turn the thermostat to a setting of 5.
   Plug the heater into a 110-volt AC outlet.
2. Attach an oxygen analyzer to the Y piece of the patient circuit. Attach a test lung to the analyzer sampling T.
3. Adjust ventilator controls as follows:

   Sensitivity = 7
   Inspiratory flow rate = 15
   Inspiratory pressure = 15
   Apnea control = off
   Air mix = off and locked

   ☐ The inspiratory pressure gauge should read 0 ± 1 cm H_2O pressure. (If the reading is off more than ± 1 cm H_2O, the gauge should be recalibrated or replaced.)
4. Set the oxygen blender control at an FI_{O_2} of 0.4.
   Attach the blender to a compressed gas source at 50 PSI.
   ☐ The blender alarm should activate.

   Comment: The pressure of both gas sources must be 40 to 60 PSI with a pressure difference between the two of no more than 10 PSI. An alarm will activate if the pressure difference becomes greater than 10 PSI or if either gas source fails, although gas from the remaining source will continue to be delivered. When you attach the blender to the gas sources, the alarm will sound until both hoses are securely attached, but this does not indicate a blender failure *unless* the alarm continues to sound after both hoses are secured.

5. Attach the blender to an oxygen source at 50 PSI.
6. Manually compress the test lung and release abruptly while observing the inspiratory pressure gauge.
   ☐ Initially the needle will deflect to -2 cm H_2O.
   ☐ Then, rather quickly, the needle should swing into the positive pressure range and should stop at 15 cm H_2O $\pm$ 1 cm H_2O as the machine cycles off.
7. Turn apnea control on (counterclockwise) one full turn.

☐ The ventilator should now cycle automatically at a constant rate.

☐ Time this rate over several cycles to assure constancy of cycling.

☐ Observe the cycling arm in the inside back of the ventilator. If the cycling arm is pushing the metal plate in toward the metal center of the ventilator, then the apnea control is determining the frequency of respiration.

Comment: If the sensitivity is set very high, this control may initiate breaths.

8. Turn apena control off.

   Remove test lung

   Connect reference spirometer to the outlet of the patient tubing in place of the test lung.

   Turn inspiratory flow to maximum.

   Trigger inflation by depressing the manual timing rod.

   Measure flow for exactly 1 minute.

   ☐ Record flow.

   _____ **LPM**

   Comment: The unrestricted flow should be at least 80 LPM. If it is not, the filters may need changing, or the Venturi gate may require cleaning.

9. Remove reference spirometer.

   Adjust ventilator controls as follows:

   Sensitivity = maximum
   Inspiratory flow rate = maximum
   Inspiratory pressure limit = minimum
   Air mix = out
   Apnea = off

10. Partially occlude the outlet of the patient tubing with your thumb.

    ☐ The ventilator should cycle off and on ("chatter") rapidly.

    Comment: This indicates that the ceramic switch is clean and functioning properly.

11. Reattach the test lung.

    Adjust inspiratory pressure limit to maximum.

    Trigger ventilator cycling by depressing the manual timing rod.

    Observe the inspiratory pressure.

    ☐ The pressure should rise to 40 cm H_2O ± 5 cm H_2O and remain constant.

    Comment: If the pressure does not reach 35 cm H_2O, there is a leak in the patient circuit, the test lung, or the high-pressure chamber of the ventilator. Check for leaks and repeat the test. If a pressure of 35 cm H_2O is still not reached, replace the ventilator. If the pressure exceeds 45 cm H$_2$O, there is a leak in the high-pressure devices requiring extensive servicing.

12. Attach reference spirometer to the expiratory outlet proximal to the Bennet spirometer. Adjust apnea control and inspiratory pressure limit so the ventilator cycles slowly (6 to 8 BPM) with tidal volumes of about 500 ml.
    ☐ Compare tidal and minute volumes as measured by the two spirometers.
    ☐ The volumes should be approximately the same. If they are not, either or both spirometers may need recalibration.

13. Attach the oxygen analyzer to the Y piece of the patient circuit. Attach a test lung to the analyzer sampling T. Allow the test lung to be ventilated for 2 minutes. Check the oxygen analyzer reading.
    ☐ The reading should agree ±5% with the oxygen setting on the blender. (If it does not, calibrate the analyzer for accuracy at 30% and 100%. Check linearity at 60%. Repeat step 13.)

14. Set the F$_{I_{O_2}}$ on the blender at 0.8.
    Allow 1 minute for a new steady state to develop.
    Check the oxygen analyzer reading.
    ☐ The reading should agree ±5% with the oxygen setting on the blender.

15. Check the temperature gauge.
    ☐ The temperature should be approximately body temperature 15 to 20 minutes after the thermostat has been turned on. Adjust setting as appropriate.

16. Prepare the ventilator for connection to the patient.
    ☐ Set all ventilator settings according to the guidelines provided.

CHAPTER 7

Initial ventilator settings

Introduction   The ventilator settings that are best for a patient must be determined by trial and error.* Fortunately, there are some guidelines about where to start so that the number of trials and the size of the errors can be kept within safe limits. Guidelines and methods for implementing them are provided.

Guidelines   Before creating a patient-ventilator system, you should attach the ventilator portion of the system to a test lung and adjust the ventilator to conform to the following guidelines:

F_{IO_2}: 1.0

V_T: 10 to 15 ml/kg

f: 10 to 15 BPM

I:E ratio: 1:2

Inspiratory flow rate: adjust as necessary to achieve the desired I:E ratio

Sensitivity: −2 cm H_2O

Sigh volume: 1.5 to 2 times the V_T every 5 minutes

Changing settings   It is anticipated that some of these settings will need revision when the patient's response to the ventilator is apparent. This response and the need for revised settings may be apparent within a few breaths or a few minutes. The patient care team must be prepared to revise the settings as needed. Making these changes is described in detail in Chapters 11 and 12.

*Depending on the settings you select, a ventilatory pattern will result. These are described in the Appendix, p. 251.

Comments on initial settings

FIO₂ The fraction of inspired oxygen may also be expressed as a percentage. For example, room air has an $F_{I_{O_2}}$ of 0.21 or 21% oxygen. On various ventilators the dial that controls $F_{I_{O_2}}$ is labelled "oxygen concentration" or "oxygen percentage." Most ventilators have an $F_{I_{O_2}}$ dial. If not, an oxygen blender should be used.

There are hazards presented by high oxygen concentrations, however. In a critically ill, newly intubated patient, use an $F_{I_{O_2}}$ of 1.0 until you can make an informed and intelligent choice of oxygen concentration based on the Pa_{O_2}. A blood gas test taken when the patient is breathing 100% oxygen also gives you an accurate alveolar-arterial gradient that is useful information. An $F_{I_{O_2}}$ of 1.0 for an hour or two probably involves little risk to the patient.

VT Tidal volume is the amount of gas mixture moved per breath. On some ventilators this is called "normal breath." On volume ventilators, control of VT is accomplished with a specific dial or by a combination of inspiratory time and flow rate. Pressure ventilators, on the other hand, deliver a VT that is dependent on the pressure setting.

Tidal volumes of 10 to 15 ml/kg may produce a higher alveolar ventilation than is needed, but the risk of atelectasis is reduced. In addition, collapsed alveoli may be reinflated. If respiratory alkalosis is produced, it may easily be controlled by addition of dead-space tubing.

A patient who has been in respiratory distress, or has vasoconstriction in response to hypoxia or to a low cardiac output, may have a large acid load to excrete. Initial settings that produce "normal" or acceptable Pa_{CO_2} and pH levels may need to be changed when the acid load is gone (in minutes to hours), or respiratory alkalosis will result.

f Frequency is commonly called respiratory rate. On some ventilators f is dialed in directly. On others it is determined by setting the expiratory time and inspiratory flow rate separately.

Dyspneic patients cannot be told to slow their respiratory rates. Initial settings on the ventilator must not only meet these patients' metabolic needs but must also meet the needs of their respiratory drives.

I:E ratio The ratio of inspiratory time to expiratory time may be dialed in directly on a few machines but is usually established by setting an inspiratory flow rate for a given minute volume or by setting both inspiratory flow rate and expiratory time for a given tidal volume.

Inspiratory time should never exceed expiratory time. During assisted (patient-assisted) ventilation, the patient should be able to control the expiratory phase. Setting the inspiratory flow rate may be complicated by the characteristics of ventilator flow and the lung compliance. Be prepared to increase the inspiratory flow rate immediately if necessary.

In emergency situations, an acceptable first setting can be determined by comparing the sound of the ventilator to your own respiratory pattern.

IFR Inspiratory flow rate is the speed with which the tidal volume is delivered. IFR is set with an uncalibrated adjustment on many of the older ventilators (Ohio 560) because the flow capabilities of the compressors were limited by the amount of back pressure in the system. On other ventilators (MA-1), IFR is controlled by a dial labelled "Peak flow rate" that indicates flow during the first part of inspiration before back pressure has accumulated. Newer ventilators (Searle VVA) are not affected as much by pressures and are calibrated in liters per minute (LPM) or liters per second (LPS).

Most pressure-cycled ventilators tend to have decelerating flow characteristics if the air-mix mode is used and constant flow characteristics if the 100% oxygen mode is used (Bird, Bennett).

Depending on the type of ventilator being used, changes in IFR may change f or the I:E ratio or may prevent delivery of tidal volume in an acceptable time.

Sensitivity Sensitivity is also called "patient effort" or "triggering effort." It is established through an uncalibrated adjustment on nearly all ventilators in current use. The sensitivity setting determines the amount of inspiratory effort required of the patient to initiate an inspiratory cycle. A high sensitivity setting will decrease the amount of patient effort required, and vice-versa. Settings for this adjustment usually range from a too-sensitive or self-cycling position to an off position or to one that requires at least -10 cm H_2O effort to cycle.

If ventilation is controlled, the patient is prevented from adjusting his ventilation with his changing metabolic needs. Control may be desired in a few unusual circumstances, but you then *must* be totally responsible for fulfilling the metabolic needs of the patient as they occur. Watch for fever, restlessness, anxiety, and other manifestations of increased need for ventilation, and be prepared to change ventilator settings. Ordinarily, the sensitivity should be set so that the patient can change his ventilation by changing his respiratory rate.

Remember, if ventilation is controlled and the patient initiates inspiratory efforts, the work of breathing, O_2 consumption, and CO_2 production will increase greatly. This situation *must* be avoided.

Expiratory resistance Expiratory resistance is also called "retard." An uncalibrated adjustment on some ventilators (MA-1) can be used to establish a resistance to exhalation, thus maintaining a higher positive pressure on the terminal airways throughout exhalation, although airway pressure returns to atmospheric levels by the end of exhalation. Retard is no longer a widely accepted ventilatory maneuver, since it can decrease cardiac output. Also, the improvement in oxygenation is less than can be attained by other maneuvers. *Expiratory resistance is not recommended.*

Sigh volume Most volume-cycled ventilators provide automatic periodic sighs. The volume of the sigh should usually be set at about 1½ to 2 times the tidal volume.

This is accomplished in some volume ventilators with a specific control. In others, the sigh volume is supplemental to the tidal volume. Most pressure-cycled ventilators do not deliver automatic sigh volumes. Increasing the volume by increasing the pressure, either by using manual controls or by inducing deep breathing with a resuscitation bag, should ideally be done every 5 to 10 minutes.

Sighs are rarely used if PEEP and large Vт's are used, as these modalities prevent alveolar collapse.

Physician's orders for mechanical ventilation

Introduction In many hospitals standing orders for patients attached to a mechanical ventilator have been established. In others, orders are written for each individual patient. Yet another method of transmitting orders is through informal consultation among team members.

Purpose The purpose of physician's orders for mechanical ventilation is the clear communication of patient goals to the nurse and therapist in the absence of the physician.

Principles Therapists and nurses should be able to adjust ventilator settings to meet patient goals without having to consult the physician each time a change needs to be made. We believe, however, that the physician should be consulted for any major changes in ventilation or patient response.

Team members should all record any changes made in ventilation as well as the effect of ventilation on the patient. These recordings should be made on one central form and be kept at the bedside.

Sample orders

GOALS FOR THE PATIENT

Keep Pa_{CO_2} between _____ and _____
Keep Pa_{O_2} between _____ and _____

Immediate orders:
   V_T _____
   f _____
   I:E ratio _____
   Maximum inspiratory pressure limit _____
   EKG monitor _____

Subsequent orders:
   Sigh volume _____
   Sigh frequency _____
   Sigh pressure limit _____
   ABGs _____
   Chest x-ray film _____
   Chest physical therapy _____
   _____
   Sedation _____
   Call MD if _____
   _____

_____ MD

Relationship of respiratory rate, tidal volume, inspiratory flow rate, expiratory time, and I:E ratio

Introduction The purpose of this section is to explain the relationship of the frequency, volume, speed, and time segments of the respiratory pattern and their implications in making and adjusting ventilator settings for optimum ventilation and patient comfort.

Rate

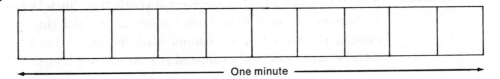

Each box represents one breath lasting 6 seconds. Therefore, f = 10.

I:E ratio

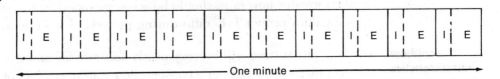

I:E ratio = 1:2, f = 10. Therefore:

Inspiratory time (I) = 2 sec/breath, 20 sec/min
Expiratory time (E) = 4 sec/breath, 40 sec/min

Tidal volume

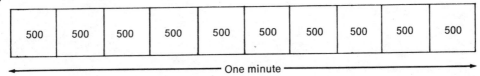

V_T = 500 ml, f = 10. Therefore:

V_E = 5000 ml or 5 L. However, the tidal volume is delivered only during the inspiratory phase. Therefore:

Flow rate

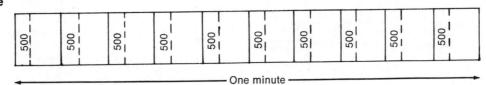

The tidal volume must be delivered in 2 seconds and the minute volume in 20 seconds. To accomplish this, the flow rate must be, at minimum, 3 times the minute volume or: 3 × 5000 ml/min = 15 LPM.

Other I:E ratios   This relationship holds true for other ratios as well. For example, for a 1:3 ratio, a flow rate equal to four times the minute ventilation would be required. For a 1:1 ratio, a flow rate equal to twice the minute ventilation would be required.

Controlled ventilation   Within the capabilities of the machine, this relationship holds true when a patient begins controlled mechanical ventilation. Such factors as accuracy of calibration, physical limitations, maintenance, and the "phantom factor"* must be considered. It is recommended, therefore, that V_T, f, IFR, and I:E ratio be monitored and evaluated at least every 2 hours.

Assisted ventilation   The patient who is being continuously ventilated in the "assist" or "assist/control" modes is establishing his own minute ventilation either continuously or intermittently and therefore must be monitored even more closely. His need for greater flow rates should be accommodated for his comfort as well as to maintain a proper I:E ratio during periods of wakefulness and activity.

Ventilator characteristics   The flow rate setting will be very nearly accurate for many of the newer volume ventilators that deliver a constant flow rate regardless of the ventilating pressures. Higher ventilating pressures may indicate a need for increasing the flow rate setting to maintain the I:E ratio.

*This term refers to those instances in which settings are changed without the knowledge of those responsible for the care of the patient.

Relationship of volume, pressure, compliance, flow, and airway resistance

Introduction The purpose of this section is to explain the relationships between lung and airway dynamics and certain ventilator parameters. These relationships should be clearly understood to ventilate optimally patients who have various types of diseases or conditions.

Basic principles
Flow and airway resistance The movement of air through airways creates friction and therefore turbulence. The more rapid the flow, the greater the friction. The narrower the airways, the greater the friction at any given flow rate. Therefore, if the flow rate is generated by spontaneous inspiration, a greater negative pressure must be created in the lung to provide a given flow rate through narrowed airways than would be required through normal airways. If the flow rate is created by a ventilator, more positive pressure is required to deliver a given flow rate through narrowed airways than through normal airways.

Volume and compliance Any container will hold a volume of gas or liquid at atmospheric pressure. If an additional volume is added, either the container must expand or the gas or liquid must be compressed. The resistance of the container to expansion is called its compliance and is expressed as liters or milliliters of volume per centimeter of water pressure (ml/cm H_2O).

The lung is normally a very compliant container (200 ml/cm H_2O). Normally the chest wall and diaphragm together are equally as compliant as the lung (200 ml/cm H_2O). These measurements are both, however, expressions of resistance to expansion. Therefore, when added together they will allow less volume per unit of pressure (100 ml/cm H_2O) than when expressed alone.

The delivery of a given volume to a lung that has lost its elastic properties will require less pressure than delivery of the same volume to a normal lung. So the lung that has lost its elastic properties is said to be more compliant.

Applied principles When a volume of gas is delivered to the patient attached to a ventilator, the pressure gauge reading will rise to a maximum inspiratory pressure (MIP) and then return to zero. The rise in pressure results from three factors:
1. Resistance to flow
    a. Magnitude of the flow rate
    b. Diameter of the airways
    c. Obstructions in the airways
2. Resistance of the lung to expansion
    a. Size of the lung
    b. Volume of gas delivered
    c. Compliance of the lung tissue

3. Resistance of the chest wall to expansion
   a. Patient position
   b. External restriction
   c. Abdominal pressure against the diaphragm
   d. Malformation of or injury to the chest wall

Dynamic compliance The relationship of the delivered volume to the total pressure required to deliver that volume is called the dynamic compliance. This value is calculated by dividing the tidal volume by the maximum inspiratory pressure and is reported as liters or milliliters per centimeter of H_2O pressure. This value is usually greater than 50 ml/cm H_2O and less than 100 ml/cm H_2O. The dynamic compliance can be used to monitor changes in pulmonary status if a baseline value is obtained after each tidal volume change. If the dynamic compliance decreases, a rather simple maneuver may be performed to isolate the airway resistance factor from the combined lung and chest wall compliance factor.

After the MIP At the end of a breath, the ventilator stops moving gas through the airways. As flow through the airways stops, the friction created by that flow disappears, causing the inspiratory pressure to drop somewhat. However, the pressure resulting from the stiffness of the lungs and chest wall (effective compliance) continues until the breath is allowed to escape.

Example If you could make a continuous recording of inspiratory pressure during mechanical ventilation, the wave form would look something like this:

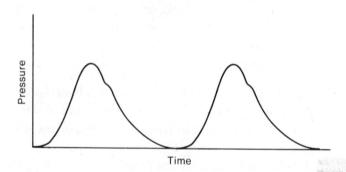

If you then measured static pressure, the wave form would look something like this:

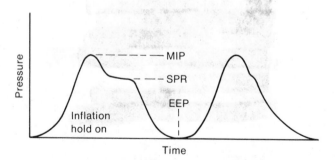

50

Static pressure The static pressure is the inspiratory pressure that persists after flow has stopped but before the breath is allowed to escape. In the usual inspiratory cycle, the static pressure is registered so briefly that it is impossible to observe.

Preparing to measure static pressure To measure static pressure, you must keep the patient's breath "trapped" in his lungs long enough to let the static pressure stabilize and be read. This brief delay in exhalation can be produced in several ways:
1. The "inflation hold" control, which some ventilators have, can be used.
2. The exhalation valve line can be deliberately kinked or occluded.
3. The exhalation port can be deliberately occluded.

Measuring static pressure
1. Allow the ventilator to start an inspiratory cycle.
2. Before the inspiratory phase is completed, occlude the expiratory line or port or activate "inflation hold."
3. Note the highest pressure (MIP) registered on the gauge.
4. The pressure will then fall slightly and stabilize—note this reading as the static pressure (SPR).
5. Allow the expiratory phase to proceed by releasing the expiratory line or port or by turning the "inflation hold" off.
6. Note the lowest pressure at the end of exhalation as the end-expiratory pressure (EEP).
7. Allow the ventilator to resume cycling as usual.
8. Record MIP, SPR, and EEP.

If you are unsure of your measurements, wait 1 minute and repeat the procedure.

Static compliance The static (or total effective) compliance is the relationship of the tidal volume to the static inspiratory pressure. The static compliance figure may be used to help find the cause for a change in dynamic compliance by separating the pressure components for airway resistance and effective compliance. A change in the dynamic compliance without a corresponding change in the static compliance indicates that there has been a change in the airway resistance. The static compliance is calculated by dividing the tidal volume by the static pressure (minus the EEP).

1. A patient has been attached to a ventilator for 3 days with an MIP of 40 cm H_2O at a tidal volume of 1 liter and a flow rate of 30 LPM.

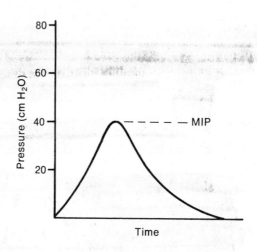

Dynamic compliance: _____

Is it normal? _____

Calculations

$$C_{dyn} = \frac{V_T}{MIP - EEP} = \frac{1\ \text{liter}}{40\ \text{cm}\ H_2O} = 0.025\ \text{L/cm}\ H_2O$$

Comment: No, it is not normal because it is less than 50 ml/cm H_2O.

2. On the fourth day the MIP rises rather suddenly to 48 cm H_2O. The static pressure is checked and found to be 20 cm H_2O.

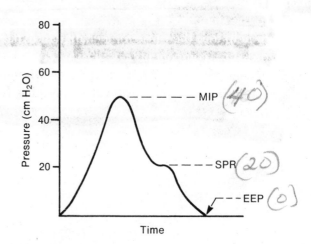

Dynamic compliance: _____

Effective compliance: _____

Airway resistance: _____

Calculations

$$C_{dyn} = \frac{V_T}{MIP - EEP} = \frac{1 \text{ liter}}{48 \text{ cm } H_2O} = 0.021 \text{ L/cm}$$

$$C_{eff} = \frac{V_T}{SPR - EEP} = \frac{1 \text{ liter}}{25 \text{ cm } H_2O} = 0.04 \text{ L/cm}$$

$$R_{aw} = \frac{MIP - SPR}{LPS} = \frac{23 \text{ cm } H_2O}{0.5 \text{ L/sec}} = 46 \text{ cm/LPS}$$

Comment: A flow rate of 30 LPM = 0.5 LPS

3. The patient is suctioned, and the endotracheal tube and ventilator tubings are found to be clear. Twenty minutes later, the MIP rises to 54 cm H_2O and the static pressure remains at 20 cm H_2O.

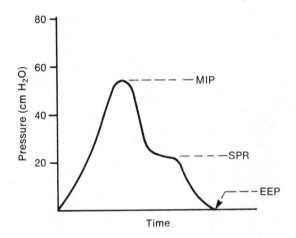

Dynamic compliance: _____

Effective compliance: _____

Airway resistance: _____

Probable cause of rise in MIP: _____

Calculations

$$C_{dyn} = \frac{V_T}{MIP - EEP} = \frac{1 \text{ liter}}{54 \text{ cm } H_2O} = 0.0185 \text{ LPM}$$

$$C_{eff} = \frac{V_T}{SPR - EEP} = \frac{1 \text{ liter}}{25 \text{ cm } H_2O} = 0.04 \text{ L/cm}$$

$$R_{aw} = \frac{MIP - SPR}{L/sec} = \frac{29 \text{ cm } H_2O}{0.5 \text{ L/sec}} = 58 \text{ cm/L/sec}$$

Comment: Increased airway resistance is probably caused by bronchospasm.

CHAPTER 8

Special problems

Hypotension and hypovolemia during mechanical ventilation

Cause Mechanical ventilation with tidal volumes over 10 ml/kg decreases cardiac output in some patients. As a result, blood pressure may fall and organ perfusion may be compromised.

Recognizing these problems These problems can be recognized in several ways. If an arterial line is in place, you will see a decrease in systolic (and, to a lesser degree, diastolic) pressure during inspiration and an increase during expiration. This phenomenon is sometimes called "respiratory swing." If the blood pressure is measured by cuff, a pulsus paradoxus will be found. If this respiratory variance in systolic blood pressure is greater than 15 mm Hg, it may have systemic effects.

Systemic effects should be evaluated by observing:
Systolic blood pressure—values below 100 may be significant
Mean arterial blood pressure—values below 70 may be associated with decreased perfusion of vital organs
Urine output—output below acceptable levels (less than 20 ml/hr) may mean compromised perfusion of the kidneys
Cerebration—evidence of obtundation or displays of confusion, hostility, or bizarre behavior may mean compromised perfusion of the brain

Comment: Most pressure monitors are capable of displaying mean arterial pressure, or it can be calculated. Either of the following formulas gives a reasonable approximation of mean arterial pressure:

$$\text{Mean} = \frac{1\,\text{systolic} + 2\,\text{diastolic}}{3}$$

Mean = Diastolic + ⅓ of pulse pressure

Management When hypotension and/or hypovolemia are confirmed in a patient being ventilated, it is important to investigate the cause. Hypotension may be caused by nonventilator-related problems, such as decreased cardiac output from heart failure. Hypovolemia may result from a previously unrecognized fluid imbalance caused by dehydration, fluid or blood losses, or sequestration of fluid.

You can sort out causes by briefly removing the ventilator from the patient. If the "respiratory swing" disappears, the swing is ventilator induced. If it continues, it is most likely caused by decreased cardiac contractility or hypovolemia and is being aggravated by the ventilator.

If the hypotension is ventilator induced, intravascular volume may have to be increased, or the tidal volume may have to be reduced. It is beyond the scope of this manual to describe the treatment of nonventilator causes of hypotension.

Pneumothorax

Patients at risk Pneumothorax occurs most frequently in patients with MIPs over 50 cm H_2O, especially if their static pressures also approach 50 cm H_2O.

Pneumothorax can be deadly in a patient with severely compromised lung function.

Be prepared If your patient requires high pressures (MIP greater than 50 cm H_2O) or is receiving PEEP, be ready to treat pneumothorax. Have the chest tube insertion tray at the patient's bedside. The suggested list of equipment for this tray appears at the end of this chapter.

Clinical clues Subtle manifestations of pneumothorax may include:
  Pleuritic pain
  Tracheal shift
  Venous distention
  Respiratory swing
  Accelerated breathing
  Breathlessness
  Gradual increase in MIP and static pressure
  Patient-ventilator asynchrony
  Subcutaneous emphysema
  Unilateral decrease in chest movement
  Unilateral decrease in breath sounds
  Hyperresonance or tympany on percussion

Signs of severe pneumothorax may include:
  Cyanosis
  Bradycardia
  Sudden rise in MIP and static pressure
  Tracheal and mediastinal shift
  Shock-like appearance
  Unconsciousness
  Blood gas results showing rapidly increasing Pa_{CO_2} and severe hypoxemia

X-ray findings may include:
  Pleural air
  Extrapleural air
  Mediastinal shift
  Tracheal shift
  Absent vascular markings in affected area
  Pulmonary vascular congestion in unaffected areas
  Depressed diaphragm with lower liver shadow or low gastric shadow

Procedure If a pneumothorax is suspected but symptoms are mild, obtain a chest x-ray film and a physician *stat*. If symptoms are acute and severe, page a physician *stat*, have a large-bore needle ready to insert, and prepare for immediate insertion of a chest tube. Also obtain a chest x-ray film *stat*.

Chest tube insertion tray   A suggested list of equipment for the insertion of a chest tube is given below. We recommend that it be assembled and stored in the ICU at all times.

1. Pleurovac or Emerson suction
2. Cutdown tray
3. Two packs sterile towels
4. Bottle of sterile water
5. Catheter tip syringe
6. 5-in-1 connector
7. Straight glass connector
8. Assortment of sterile gloves
9. Heimlich valve
10. Right angle thoracic catheters (32 and 34)
11. Trocar catheters (28, 32, 36)
12. Thoracic catheters (28, 32, 36, 40)
13. Bottle of Betadine solution
14. 10 sterile 4 × 4s
15. Spinal needles (18, 20, 22)
16. Tape (1 and 2 inch)
17. Alcohol swabs
18. 00 and 000 silk
19. Scalpel blade (11)
20. 20 ml 1% lidocaine

PART TWO

Managing the patient-ventilator system

CHAPTER 9

Introduction to managing the system

Introduction Once the patient and the ventilator are connected, you have created a new system. The main purpose of this system is to regulate the patient's blood gases. This can be achieved with minimum risk and discomfort to the patient.

Goals for the patient If you are taking care of a patient attached to a ventilator your goals are to:
Maintain the patient's Pa_{O_2} within safe limits
Maintain the patient's pH and Pa_{CO_2} as close to his normal as possible
Detect patient problems early
Detect ventilator problems early
Keep the patient comfortable

Basic rules Experience has shown that these goals are easier to achieve if you observe some basic rules:
Never leave the system unattended. A nurse or therapist should be near and watching the system constantly.
Monitor the system at regular intervals. Detect problems when they first arise and are easier to correct.
Anticipate your response to problems. Know your next move. When you monitor the patient, ask yourself, "What if . . . ?"

Part II Part II will describe how to:
Be prepared
Adjust the $F_{I_{O_2}}$
Maintain the desired pH and Pa_{CO_2}
Monitor the patient and troubleshoot
Monitor the ventilator and troubleshoot
Bag the patient
Suction the airway
Keep the patient comfortable
Move secretions into the upper airway
Prevent deconditioning
Administer PEEP therapy
Wean the patient

CHAPTER 10

Be prepared

Develop and maintain skills

Becoming prepared means learning certain skills. The chapters that follow are designed to help you learn these skills.

If you have not recently or frequently managed a patient attached to a ventilator, it is recommended that you practice your skills using the various exercises provided in Part III of this book.

Be near

Being prepared also means being close enough to the patient to detect problems and solve them quickly. For this reason we consider it essential that a nurse or a therapist remain within immediate reach of the patient-ventilator system at all times.

Know goals and strategy

Being prepared means having the immediate goals of maintenance of the Pa_{O_2} and pH clearly in mind. In addition, the health care team must decide what the overall goals of ventilation are. Making this decision requires knowing:

    The initial reason for mechanical ventilation

    The anticipated duration of ventilation

    The criteria by which successful achievement of goals will be recognized

Assemble tools

Being prepared means having your tools ready and immediately available at the bedside. Here is the list of equipment needed for maintaining continuous ventilation:

1. ECG monitor
2. Suction source, catheters, gloves, and tonsil tip sucker
3. Manual resuscitation bag
4. Syringe appropriate for cuff size
5. Rubber-tipped clamp
6. Extra endotracheal tube appropriate for patient
7. Extra connectors, adaptors, and dead-space tubing
8. O_2 analyzer
9. Spirometer
10. Stethoscope
11. Sterile distilled water

12. Magic slate or other means of communication
13. ABG determination capability
14. Rubber test lung

CHAPTER 11

Adjusting the $F_{I_{O_2}}$

Goals   In most patients, the Pa_{O_2} should be maintained between 60 mm and 100 mm Hg.

Principle $F_{I_{O_2}}$ is adjusted to avoid the hazards of both hypoxemia and oxygen toxicity. Hypoxemia (Pa_{O_2} less than 55 mm Hg) is a more immediate hazard than O_2 toxicity. Consequently, accepted practice is to start with a high $F_{I_{O_2}}$ (1.0), check the Pa_{O_2}, and adjust the $F_{I_{O_2}}$ downward to achieve the Pa_{O_2} goal.

Basic rule   If the current $F_{I_{O_2}}$ does not result in a Pa_{O_2} greater than 60 mm Hg, increase $F_{I_{O_2}}$ to 1.0 and follow the procedure below:

Procedure
1. Initiate ventilation with an $F_{I_{O_2}}$ of 1.0.
2. Wait 20 minutes for Pa_{O_2} to stabilize.
3. Measure ABGs.
4. Adjust $F_{I_{O_2}}$ downward in steps to achieve a Pa_{O_2} of 60 to 100 mm Hg.
   a. *If* the Pa_{O_2} is greater than 300, *then* drop $F_{I_{O_2}}$ by steps of 0.20.
   b. *If* the Pa_{O_2} is 150 to 300, *then* drop $F_{I_{O_2}}$ by steps of 0.10.
   c. *If* the Pa_{O_2} is 100 to 150, *then* drop $F_{I_{O_2}}$ by steps of 0.05.
5. Recheck the Pa_{O_2} 20 minutes after each downward adjustment.

Comments   Some practitioners consider the suggested steps too cautious. Indeed, in many instances they may be. However, you cannot accurately predict the change in Pa_{O_2} that will result from a decrease in $F_{I_{O_2}}$. Therefore, in an unstable patient with an unknown history, we suggest a cautious approach.

Consider the use of PEEP if an $F_{I_{O_2}}$ greater than 0.5 is required to maintain a Pa_{O_2} greater than 60 mm Hg.

COPD patients may be accustomed to a Pa_{O_2} below 55 mm Hg.

Pa_{O_2} is a reflection of lung function, not of tissue oxygenation. Patients with a low hemoglobin or low cardiac output will have a decrease in oxygen delivery to the tissues. Evaluation and support of hemoglobin and cardiac function should be considered in improving oxygen transport.

In very sick patients, it is difficult to increase the Pa_{O_2} by increasing FI_{O_2}. More dramatic improvement depends on therapy that reverses abnormalities. Such therapy includes clearing the airways, treating atelectasis, and increasing cardiac output.

CHAPTER 12

Maintaining the desired pH and Pa_{CO_2}

Goals Maintenance of a pH near normal
Maintenance of a Pa_{CO_2} near normal for the patient

Principle The ventilator gives you control over the patient's Pa_{CO_2}. When you increase the rate or depth of respiration, you "blow off" CO_2, and Pa_{CO_2} decreases. When the Pa_{CO_2} decreases, pH increases. Decreasing the rate or tidal volume has the opposite effect. Therefore, be prepared to adjust the rate and depth of respiration to keep the pH near normal. However, severe metabolic acidosis or alkalosis should *not* be treated by manipulating Pa_{CO_2} *only*.

pH goals Arterial pH is normally about 7.40. How close to normal should the pH be kept in a ventilator patient? If you want the patient to relax and let the ventilator do all the work, then aim for a pH around 7.45. Mild alkalosis (7.43 to 7.46) decreases respiratory drive and permits easier control of ventilation. However, realize that pH above 7.47 may cause arrhythmias, decreased cardiac output, seizures, and other problems.

If the patient has COPD, he may be accustomed to a Pa_{CO_2} above normal and a pH slightly below 7.40. Adjust ventilation in these patients to achieve a pH around 7.37. This will make weaning easier.

If the patient has metabolic acidosis, do not attempt to restore normal pH by hyperventilation only. Treat the cause of metabolic acidosis if possible, or use bicarbonate.

Procedure A: a simple approach
1. Adjust the ventilator settings to achieve the goals described in Chapter 7.
2. Wait 20 minutes for a steady state to be reached.
3. Measure arterial blood gases.
4. Measure or calculate minute ventilation ($\dot{V}_E$).
5. Assume the following simple inverse relationship between existing and future values:

$$\dot{V}_E \cdot Pa_{CO_2} = \dot{V}_E' \cdot Pa_{CO_2}'$$

or

$$V_T \cdot f \cdot Pa_{CO_2} = V_T' \cdot f' \cdot Pa_{CO_2}'$$

Calculate the minute ventilation to achieve the desired Pa_{CO_2}.

6. In adjusting for the new $\dot{V}_E$, we assume you had a minimum V_T of 10 ml/kg of body weight. Increase as needed up to 15 ml/kg, *then* adjust f to achieve the desired $\dot{V}_E$.

7. Recheck arterial blood gas levels in 20 minutes.

8. Be prepared to provide an even larger $\dot{V}_E$ than the formula suggests.

Example for procedure A

Patient weight = 70 kg
    Current V_T = 840 ml (12 ml/kg)
                f = 14
Current Pa_{CO_2} = 45 mm Hg

This Pa_{CO_2} is higher than you wish, based on your pH goal. You decide that a more desirable Pa_{CO_2} is 35 mm Hg. You decide to increase the V_T rather than the f. Your formula is:

$$V_T \cdot f \cdot Pa_{CO_2} = V_T' \cdot f \cdot Pa_{CO_2}'$$

Therefore:

$$840 \cdot 14 \cdot 45 = V_T' \cdot 14 \cdot 35$$

    or

$$529{,}200 = V_T' \cdot 490$$
$$V_T = 1080 \text{ ml } (15.4 \text{ ml/kg})$$

(') stands for the new or desired value.

Please refer to p. 72 for a detailed explanation of how to use this formula if it is still not clear.

Procedure B: adjusting for estimated dead space

The formula suggested above does not recognize the role of dead space. The dead space of the ventilator and tubing can usually be estimated. The dead space of a normal person is about 2 ml/kg of body weight. The formula is:

$$(V_T - V_{D_{anat}} - V_{D_{added}}) \cdot f \cdot Pa_{CO_2} = (V_T' - V_{D_{anat}} - V_{D_{added}}') \cdot f' \cdot Pa_{CO_2}'$$

Please refer to p. 73 for a detailed explanation of how to use this formula.

Which setting to change

You must decide which setting is most appropriate to change. If respiratory *alkalosis* exists:

    V_T should not be decreased below the desired volume of 10 to 15 ml/kg.
    Changing f below 10 to 15 BPM usually causes the patient to be uncomfortable. 150 cc
Therefore, adding dead space is often the most appropriate change.

If respiratory *acidosis* exists:

    V_T should be increased to 15 ml/kg (or higher if MIPs permit).
    f can be increased.
    Excess dead-space tubing may be removed, but a small piece should be left in place for easier airway management.

Clinical guidelines   To review and summarize what has been discussed, we offer the following guidelines:

1. Measure arterial blood gases.
2. Measure minute ventilation.
3. Using the following formula, calculate the minute ventilation required to achieve a Pa_{CO_2} of about 35 mm Hg in patients who do not have chronic lung disease:

$$V_T \cdot f \cdot Pa_{CO_2} = V_T{}' \cdot f' \cdot Pa_{CO_2}{}'$$

4. Adjust the tidal volume from 10 to 15 ml/kg as needed; then adjust the respiratory rate, if necessary, to change the minute ventilation.
5. Recheck the blood gas levels in about 20 minutes. *Do not wait hours to recheck the blood gases.*

Achieving the desired Pa$_{CO_2}$: one way of thinking about it

Introduction

We will now discuss further the manipulation of the ventilator to achieve a desired Pa$_{CO_2}$. We will present the concepts and several examples of how to estimate the changes in settings that may be required for your particular patient.

Patient-controlled ventilation

If the patient is alert and initiating breaths, the easiest way to achieve a relatively constant and appropriate Pa$_{CO_2}$ is to *assist* ventilation. The patient initiates each breath, and the ventilator then turns on and delivers a tidal volume determined by where *you* set the dials. We recommend a tidal volume of 10 to 15 ml/kg. The patient—if his respiratory center is functioning—will then adjust his respiratory rate to get the Pa$_{CO_2}$ that his respiratory center "wants." In addition, we recommend setting a "backup" rate of 10 BPM.

If you set the ventilator to deliver a small tidal volume, the patient will breathe at a faster rate. If you deliver a large tidal volume (which is the usual practice), the respiratory rate will slow. The patient can thus adjust his minute ventilation continuously by varying his respiratory rate.

Unless you have a patient with a respiratory center severely depressed from drugs or trauma, this is the ideal way to ventilate.

Controlled ventilation

Sometimes it is necessary to control ventilation—for example, in the cases of drug overdose or severe depression of the respiratory center because of trauma or cerebral bleeding. In these situations, you have to select and set a minute ventilation by setting both tidal volume and frequency to keep Pa$_{CO_2}$ within an acceptable range.

This does not mean that the patient is not allowed to initiate breaths; rather it means that he is unable to do so for some reason.

How to think about controlling ventilation

These important variables relate to each other and to CO_2 production:

$$Pa_{CO_2} \sim \frac{CO_2 \text{ production}}{\text{Alveolar ventilation}}$$

For example, in a normal, resting, 70 kg man, the corresponding values would be:

$$40 \text{ mm Hg} \sim \frac{200 \text{ ml/min}}{5 \text{ LPM}}$$

This equation states that the arterial Pa$_{CO_2}$ is *directly* related to the rate of CO_2 production and inversely related to the rate of alveolar ventilation. The Pa$_{CO_2}$ is normally near 40 mm Hg. For example, if you run up stairs, you increase your rate of CO_2 production, but your Pa$_{CO_2}$ stays at 40 because you also increase your rate of alveolar ventilation. That is why you are puffing when you reach the top of the stairs. Patients may not be able to increase their rates of ventilation (as in the drug overdose example), so you must set those rates to meet their needs, which will vary with their metabolic rates.

69

Alveolar ventilation vs minute ventilation

How does alveolar ventilation differ from minute ventilation? Alveolar ventilation ($\dot{V}_A$) is the minute ventilation ($\dot{V}_E$) minus the dead space (V_D). Since dead space is part of each tidal volume, the formula is:

$$\dot{V}_A = (V_T - V_D) \times f$$

EXAMPLE: $4500 \text{ ml} = (600 \text{ ml} - 150 \text{ ml}) \times 10$

Dead space

Dead space is the portion of the tidal volume that does not participate in gas exchange (about one third of each tidal volume or 2 ml/kg of tidal volume). We can measure it, but not conveniently. We can measure minute ventilation conveniently with a simple, inexpensive, bedside spirometer.

In addition to being difficult to measure, the amount of dead space varies with:

The amount of connecting tubing in the system
The size of the tidal volume
The nature of the lung disease
The circulatory status of the patient

So for practical purposes, we use the minute ventilation as a guide to achieve the desired Pa_{CO_2}.

Most disease states result in an increase in dead space, so you usually have to provide a larger minute ventilation than you would for a normal individual.

$$Pa_{CO_2} (40 \text{ mm Hg}) \sim \frac{CO_2 \text{ production } (200 \text{ ml/min})}{\text{Alveolar ventilation } (5 \text{ LPM})}$$

You see that in a normal individual, if you double alveolar ventilation, you halve the Pa_{CO_2}.

$$Pa_{CO_2} (20 \text{ mm Hg}) \sim \frac{CO_2 \text{ production } (200 \text{ ml/min})}{\text{Alveolar ventilation } (10 \text{ LPM})}$$

An example

Let's take an example in a patient. You have begun to ventilate a barbiturate-overdose patient. Twenty minutes later a blood gas check reveals a Pa_{CO_2} of 60 mm Hg. The measured minute ventilation is 6.0 LPM. The patient is not agitated, he is not fighting the ventilator, and he is not febrile—that is, CO_2 production is not acutely elevated. These facts can be established by simple physical examination of the patient.

You decide you want the Pa_{CO_2} to be 30 to 35 mm Hg. You could therefore double the minute ventilation to 12 LPM. Theoretically this should halve the Pa_{CO_2}, but you have to check the blood gas levels after the change. Why? Because you do not know the amount of dead space or the rate of alveolar ventilation. You may not cut the Pa_{CO_2} in half if the dead space volume is large.

Adjusting the ventilator Should you increase the respiratory rate or the tidal volume in order to increase the ventilation? We recommend using a tidal volume of 10 to 15 ml/kg in almost all ventilator patients. Once this volume is achieved, adjusting the respiratory rate is the simplest way to adjust the Pa_{CO_2}.

You should also observe the amount of dead-space tubing in the ventilator circuit. Decreasing external dead space also contributes to solving your problem. However, keeping a small piece of dead space tubing in the circuit makes airway management more comfortable for the patient and easier for you.

In summary $$Pa_{CO_2} \sim \frac{CO_2 \text{ production}}{\text{Alveolar ventilation}}$$

CO_2 production may change rapidly if the metabolic activity of the patient changes.

Alveolar ventilation may change if: (1) dead space volume changes, (2) you are using a pressure ventilator and the lung compliance changes, or (3) the patient is sedated and has a depressed respiratory rate.

Minute ventilation does not relate in a precise arithmetic way to Pa_{CO_2} because it is alveolar ventilation that determines Pa_{CO_2}.

In clinical practice we do not need very precise control of the Pa_{CO_2}, so we can use minute ventilation as a guide if we recognize that disease states invariably increase the dead space and the required minute ventilation.

Clinical guidelines For practical purposes, follow these steps when you adjust minute ventilation:

1. Measure arterial blood gases.
2. Measure minute ventilation.
3. Assume an inverse relationship between Pa_{CO_2} and $\dot{V}_E$. Calculate the minute ventilation required to achieve a Pa_{CO_2} of 30 to 35 mm Hg with a pH of ~7.45.
4. Ensure a tidal volume of 10 to 15 ml/kg. Then adjust respiratory rate if necessary.
5. If both rate and volume are at optimal settings, consider the use of more or less dead-space tubing.
6. Recheck blood gas levels in 20 minutes.

Procedure A: a simple approach

The problem Your patient is undergoing continuous controlled ventilation. You want to keep his Pa_{CO_2} at 35 mm Hg (and pH ~ 7.45). The latest blood gas analysis shows: $Pa_{CO_2} = 50$ (pH ~ 7.30). You realize that you must increase the ventilation, but *how much* should you increase it and *how?*

Solution You can approximate the new minute volume you want by using one simple formula:

$$\dot{V}_E' = \frac{Pa_{CO_2} \times \dot{V}_E}{Pa_{CO_2}'} \qquad \text{(This formula is easier for us nonalgebraic people.)}$$

In which:

$\dot{V}_E$ = minute ventilation
Pa_{CO_2} = measured arterial Pa_{CO_2}
$'$ = prime (new or desired value)

Rationale $\dot{V}_E' = \frac{Pa_{CO_2} \times \dot{V}_E}{Pa_{CO_2}'} \qquad (or: \dot{V}_E \cdot Pa_{CO_2} = \dot{V}_E' \cdot Pa_{CO_2}')$

The level of Pa_{CO_2} in the arterial blood is inversely proportional to minute ventilation. If minute ventilation doubles, theoretically Pa_{CO_2} is halved. Hence you can approximate the required $\dot{V}_E$ for a desired Pa_{CO_2}, if you know current Pa_{CO_2} and $\dot{V}_E$.

Steps 1. Measure $\dot{V}_E$
Measure V_T
Measure f
Multiply $V_T \times f$ to solve for $\dot{V}_E$

EXAMPLE: $V_T = 700$
$f = 12$
$\dot{V}_E = 700 \times 12$

2. Measure Pa_{CO_2}
3. Decide desired Pa_{CO_2}
4. Solve for new $\dot{V}_E$

Example 1

$V_T = 700$ ml   Current $Pa_{CO_2} = 50$ mm Hg
$f = 12$ Desired $Pa_{CO_2} = 35$ mm Hg
$\dot{V}_E = 8400$ ml (8.4 L)

$$\dot{V}_E' = \frac{Pa_{CO_2} \times \dot{V}_E}{Pa_{CO_2}'}$$

$$\dot{V}_E' = \frac{50 \times 8400}{35}$$

$$\dot{V}_E' = \frac{420,000}{35}$$

$$\dot{V}_E' = 12,000 \text{ ml or } 12 \text{ L}$$

Example 2

$V_T = 100$
$f = 14$
$\dot{V}_E = 15{,}400 \text{ ml} (15.4 \text{ L})$

Current $Pa_{CO_2} = 28$ mm Hg
Desired $Pa_{CO_2} = 40$ mm Hg

$$\dot{V}_E' = \frac{Pa_{CO_2} \times \dot{V}_E}{Pa_{CO_2}'}$$

$$\dot{V}_E' = \frac{28 \times 15{,}400}{40}$$

$$\dot{V}_E' = \frac{431{,}200}{40'}$$

$$\dot{V}_E' = 10{,}780 \text{ ml or } 10.8 \text{ L}$$

Procedure B: adjusting for estimated dead space

Comment This formula is somewhat more complex because it recognizes the role that dead space plays in the determination of alveolar ventilation and also, therefore, in Pa_{CO_2}. The dead space of the ventilator and tubing can usually be estimated. The dead space of a normal person is about 2 ml/kg.

The formula The formula is:

$$(V_T - V_{D_{anat}} - V_{D_{added}}) \cdot f \cdot Pa_{CO_2} = (V_T' - V_{D_{anat}} - V_{D_{added}}') \cdot f \cdot Pa_{CO_2}'$$

Therefore, it is clear that Pa_{CO_2} can be altered by: (1) changing V_T, (2) changing V_D, or (3) changing f.

Example 1

Assume the following situation:

$Wt = 100$ kg
$V_T = 1000$ ml
$f = 15$
Desired $Pa_{CO_2} = 40$

$V_{D_{anat}} = 200$ ml
$V_{D_{added}} = 0$
Measured $Pa_{CO_2} = \underline{20 \text{ mm Hg}}$

How to change f

$(V_T - V_{D_{anat}} - V_{D_{added}}) \cdot f \cdot Pa_{CO_2} = (V_T - V_{D_{anat}} - V_{D_{added}}) \cdot f' \cdot Pa_{CO_2}'$
$(1000 - 200 - 0) \cdot 15 \cdot 20 = (1000 - 200 - 0) \cdot f' \cdot 40$
$(800) \cdot 15 \cdot 20 = (800) \; f' \cdot 40$
$240{,}000 = 32{,}000 \; f'$
$\frac{240}{32}$ $7.5 = f'$

This example illustrates that changing *only* f will result in an f lower than most patients can tolerate. Either V_T or V_D should be changed instead (or as well) to maintain $f \sim 10$ while achieving the desired Pa_{CO_2}.

How to change V_T

$$(V_T - V_{D_{anat}} - V_{D_{added}}) \cdot f \cdot Pa_{CO_2} = (V_T' - V_{D_{anat}} - V_{D_{added}}) \cdot f \cdot Pa_{CO_2}'$$
$$(1000 - 200 - 0) \cdot 15 \cdot 20 = (V_T' - 200 - 0) \cdot 15 \cdot 40$$
$$(800) \cdot 15 \cdot 20 = (V_T' - 200 - 0) \cdot 15 \cdot 40$$
$$240,000 = 600 \ V_T' - 120,000$$
$$360,000 = 600 \ V_T'$$
$$800 = V_T'$$

Although this change in V_T will achieve a Pa_{CO_2} close to the desired 40, we recommend using a V_T of at least 10 ml/kg. Therefore, other settings should be changed.

How to change $V_{D_{added}}$

$$(V_T - V_{D_{anat}} - V_{D_{added}}) \cdot f \cdot Pa_{CO_2} = (V_T - V_{D_{anat}} - V_{D_{added}}') \cdot f \cdot Pa_{CO_2}'$$
$$(1000 - 200 - 0) \cdot 15 \cdot 20 = (1000 - 200 - V_{D_{added}}') \cdot 15 \cdot 40$$
$$(800) \cdot 15 \cdot 20 = (800 - V_{D_{added}}') \cdot 15 \cdot 40$$
$$240,000 = 480,000 - 600 \ V_{D_{added}}'$$
$$240,000 = 600 \ V_{D_{added}}'$$
$$400 = V_{D_{added}}'$$

This is an appropriate change to make. V_T is maintained at 10 ml/kg and f at 15. The Pa_{CO_2} would be in the range of 40.

How to change $V_{D_{added}}$ and f

$$(V_T - V_{D_{anat}} - V_{D_{added}}) \cdot f \cdot Pa_{CO_2} = (V_T - V_{D_{anat}} - V_{D_{added}}') \cdot f' \cdot Pa_{CO_2}'$$

Select a desired f'. We have selected an f' of 10.

$$(1000 - 200 - 0) \cdot 15 \cdot 20 = (1000 - 200 - V_{D_{added}}') \cdot 10 \cdot 40$$
$$(800) \cdot 15 \cdot 20 = (800 - V_{D_{added}}') \cdot 10 \cdot 40$$
$$240,000 = 320,000 - 400 \ V_{D_{added}}'$$
$$80,000 = 400 \ V_{D_{added}}'$$
$$200 \ ml = V_{D_{added}}'$$

This is an appropriate change to make.

Example 2

Assume the following situation:

Wt = 80 kg	$V_{D_{anat}}$ = 160 ml
V_T = 800 ml	$V_{D_{added}}$ = 30 ml
f = 10	Measured Pa_{CO_2} = 60 mm Hg
Desired Pa_{CO_2} = 40	

How to change f

$$(V_T - V_{D_{anat}} - V_{D_{added}}) \cdot f \cdot Pa_{CO_2} = (V_T - V_{D_{anat}} - V_{D_{added}}) \cdot f' \cdot Pa_{CO_2}'$$
$$(800 - 160 - 30) \cdot 10 \cdot 60 = (800 - 160 - 30) \cdot f' \cdot 40$$
$$(600) \cdot 10 \cdot 60 = (610) \cdot f' \cdot 40$$
$$366,000 = 24,400 \ f'$$
$$15 = f'$$

This is an appropriate change to make. However, the patient should be evaluated for the cause of the elevated Pa_{CO_2}. Perhaps the V_T should be greater.

How to change V_T

$$(V_T - V_{D_{anat}} - V_{D_{added}}) \cdot f \cdot Pa_{CO_2} = (V_T' - V_{D_{anat}} - V_{D_{added}}) \cdot f \cdot Pa_{CO_2}'$$
$$(800 - 160 - 30) \cdot 10 \cdot 60 = (V_T' - 160 - 30) \cdot 10 \cdot 40$$
$$610 \cdot 10 \cdot 60 = (V_T' - 190) \cdot 10 \cdot 40$$
$$366,000 = 400 \, V_T' - 76,000$$
$$442,000 = 400 \, V_T'$$
$$1105 \text{ ml} = V_T'$$

This is an appropriate change to make.

How to change $V_{D_{added}}$

$$(V_T - V_{D_{anat}} - V_{D_{added}}) \cdot f \cdot Pa_{CO_2} = (V_T - V_{D_{anat}} - V_{D_{added}}') \cdot f \cdot Pa_{CO_2}'$$
$$(800 - 160 - 30) \cdot 10 \cdot 60 = (800 - 160 - V_{D_{added}}') \cdot 10 \cdot 40$$
$$(610) \cdot 10 \cdot 60 = (640 - V_{D_{added}}') \cdot 10 \cdot 40$$
$$366,000 = 256,000 - 400 \, V_{D_{added}}'$$
$$110,000 = V_{D_{added}}'$$
$$-275 = V_{D_{added}}'$$

This is obviously not possible, as only 30 ml of V_D are in the circuit. Other settings must be changed.

How to change $V_{D_{added}}$ and f

$$(V_T - V_{D_{anat}} - V_{D_{added}}) \cdot f \cdot Pa_{CO_2} = (V_T - V_{D_{anat}} - V_{D_{added}}') \cdot f' \cdot Pa_{CO_2}'$$
$$(800 - 160 - 30) \cdot 10 \cdot 60 = (800 - 160 - V_{D_{added}}') \cdot f' \cdot 40$$
$$(610) \cdot 10 \cdot 60 = (800 - 160 - 0) \cdot f' \cdot 40$$
$$366,000 = 25,600 \, f'$$
$$14 = f'$$
$$0 = V_{D_{added}}$$

This is an appropriate change to make. 30 ml of V_D was removed, and f should be increased to 14.

Assumptions and pitfalls

The methods described in the preceding pages are intended to reduce guesswork involved in adjusting a ventilator. If you use the formulas as directed, you should find it easier to get close to the desired Pa_{CO_2}. However, the method is not perfect. Be prepared for some situations that do not go "according to the book." What accounts for such situations? You must realize that the formulas are based on two important assumptions. It is assumed that: (1) metabolic rate does not change, and (2) physiologic dead space does not change.

If the metabolic rate increases, more CO_2 is produced. When more CO_2 is produced, the alveolar ventilation must be increased or CO_2 will accumulate in the blood (and the Pa_{CO_2} will rise). The reverse is also true. For example, consider a patient who is struggling because he is not satisfied by the tidal volume. If you increase the tidal volume, he may relax, and his metabolic rate will be decreased. His Pa_{CO_2} will drop more than you would expect from the increased ventilation alone. Be prepared to make allowances for Pa_{CO_2} changes that can result from struggling, fever, or sedation.

Also be prepared to make allowances for variations in physiologic dead space. Although 2 ml/kg is a useful rule of thumb for estimating anatomic dead space, physiologic dead space varies from person to person and moment to moment. Certain diseases, like emphysema, are associated with abnormally large physiologic dead space. In some patients, the dead space will seem to change from one ventilator setting to another as airways open up or atelectatic segments clear. Be prepared to recognize such changes when they occur.

Finally, still other factors, such as compression of gas in ventilator tubing, will produce results that seem at variance with calculations. Do not be discouraged by these extra problems. They merely require some "fine tuning." The two formulas still will help you make the big adjustments.

CHAPTER 13

Monitoring the patient

Goal The goal of monitoring is to detect problems early when they are easier to correct.

Principle The patient part of the patient-ventilator system should be checked in a systematic way at least hourly. The unstable patient may require continuous monitoring and assessment. The monitoring routine should distinguish between conditions that simply need to be checked ("Are things still ok?") and those that need to be measured and recorded.

Review your routine We recommend that you examine your present method of monitoring the patient to ensure that mechanisms for observation and recording are adequate, clearly understood, and followed by all team members.

We have previously recommended that a nurse or a therapist be within sight and sound of every patient being ventilated. This should permit frequent assessment of the patient. A systematic assessment routine should be established for ventilator patients in your particular intensive care unit. Each team member should learn and use the same routine procedures, which may include maintaining a check sheet, a poster, or other devices to decrease reliance on memory alone.

Scanning and checking With a nurse close to each ventilator patient, it should be possible to monitor some aspects of the patient's condition almost continuously. At all times the patient should be attached to a cardiac monitor with alarm limits set. In addition, the nurse should scan continuously for clinical signs and symptoms. Periodically, the team members should direct conscious attention to evaluation, measurement, and recording of data to ensure early recognition of signs and symptoms that may indicate problems.

Evaluating, measuring, recording

What to evaluate	*How often*
Vital signs	
Blood pressure	Every 1-4 hours
Presence of respiratory swing	With each blood pressure reading
Heart rate and rhythm	Every hour
Urinary output	Every hour or voiding

Evaluating, measuring, recording (cont'd)	*What to evaluate*	*How often*
	Temperature	Every 1-4 hours
	Respiratory rate	Every hour
	Weight	Daily
	Physical examination	
	Synchrony with the ventilator	Every hour
	Air leak from endotracheal tube	Every hour
	Breath sounds	Every 1-4 hours
	Subcutaneous emphysema	Every 1-4 hours
	Skin temperature and moisture	Every 1-4 hours
	Pulses	Every hour
	Character of secretions	With every suctioning
	Gastric distention	Every 1-4 hours
	Air leak via chest tube	Every hour
	Laboratory work and x-ray film	
	Arterial blood gases	With every change in ventilator setting
		With any unexplained or not easily correctable patient change
	Serum potassium	Daily or more often
	Serum sodium	Twice weekly or more often
	Chest x-ray films	Daily or more often
	Patient behavior	
	Anxiety, fear	Every hour
	Restlessness, agitation	Every hour
	Confusion, disorientation, inappropriate behavior	Every hour
	Somnolence, obtundation	Every hour
	Dyspnea	Every hour
	Headache	Every hour or when awake
	Twitching, tetany, convulsions	Every hour
	Asterixis	Every hour

CHAPTER 14

Troubleshooting: clues the patient offers

Introduction When routine monitoring of the patient discloses a warning sign or symptom, a search for an emerging problem should begin. This chapter offers suggestions for identifying and correcting such problems.

Nonventilator-related problems Connecting a patient to a ventilator does not protect him from the problems of the medical or surgical patient, for example, myocardial infarction, pulmonary embolus, gastrointestinal (GI) bleeding, sepsis. In order words, you should apply your clinical experience with nonventilator patients to the analysis of the problems of ventilator patients. However, you must augment this experience with knowledge of problems that relate to the use of mechanical ventilation.

Ventilator-related problems This chapter will concentrate on the problems related to mechanical ventilation. A table of clues, possible problems, and advice is offered. Throughout that table you will notice some recurring possible problems, including pneumothorax, hypoxia, abnormal Pa_{CO_2}, obstruction of the right main stem bronchus, decreased venous return, and the variety of ways in which air leaks out of the patient-ventilator system. A brief review of these recurring problems is in order.

Pneumothorax The risk of pneumothorax increases if maximum inspiratory pressures are high (over 50 cm H_2O). Further impairment of lung function may be rapid and severe. The treatment—insertion of a chest tube—is simple and specific. The possibility of pneumothorax should be considered early in evaluating almost any deterioration in the condition of a patient being ventilated.

Abnormalities of Pa_{O_2} and Pa_{CO_2} The early signs of hypoxia are varied and are *not specific*. The signs of abnormal Pa_{CO_2} and pH are also varied and are *not specific*. Therefore, when in doubt, check the blood gas levels.

Obstruction of the right main stem bronchus When an endotracheal tube is displaced and slips down the trachea too far, the tube enters the right main stem bronchus *and* occludes the left main stem bronchus. As a result, the right lung is overventilated (and at risk of pneumothorax). Also, the airway to the left lung is completely obstructed. Further impairment of lung function follows. The patient's condition deteriorates and the ventilator becomes difficult to regulate. The treatment is simple and specific: reposition the tube.

Decreased venous return Positive-pressure ventilation impedes venous return. This may reduce cardiac output and lower blood pressure—especially during the inspiratory phase. The body attempts to compensate for these developments by retaining fluid and expanding blood volume. However, this compensation proceeds slowly. If hypotension becomes serious, it may be necessary to augment the intravascular volume rapidly with intravenous fluids or blood.

Leaks Effective positive-pressure ventilation depends on maintaining an airtight connection between the ventilator and the patient's lungs. A leak can result in failure to ventilate the lungs adequately. If the patient does not seem to be getting enough to breathe, consider a leak somewhere in the system.

Obstructions Failure to ventilate also can be caused by plugs, kinks, and other obstructions. Tubings can be kinked or crimped behind a recently moved bed or bedside stand. Patient circuits may be incorrectly assembled, creating inappropriate ventilation.

Resets If you are monitoring a patient attached to a ventilator, you tend to assume that all adjustments of the controls and settings come to your attention. Yet experience has shown that this is not always true. Dials are sometimes accidentally moved and reset. Settings are sometimes changed by another member of the team without notifying you. If things are not going well, consider the possibility that the settings have been adjusted without your knowledge.

Check the system and settings In the following tables, you will often be advised to "check the patient-ventilator system and settings." This means double-check for leaks, obstructions, resets, and other common problems.

Troubleshooting tables for "clues the patient offers"

For clues related to:	See:
Patient behaviors	Table 4
Vital signs	Table 5
Physical examination	Table 6
Laboratory work and x-ray film	Table 7

Table 4 Patient behaviors

Clue	Possible problems	Advice
Mental status		
Anxiety, fear	Response to new environment or to being ventilated	Reassure, alleviate fears; explain safeguards
	$\downarrow Pa_{O_2}$	Check patient-ventilator system; if not easily alleviated, obtain and evaluate ABGs
Restlessness, agitation	$\downarrow Pa_{O_2}$, $\downarrow Pa_{CO_2}$	Check patient-ventilator system; if not easily corrected, obtain and evaluate ABGs
	Pain	Check for pain medication needs
Confusion, disorientation, inappropriate behavior	$\downarrow Pa_{O_2}$	Check patient-ventilator system
		Check $F_{I_{O_2}}$ setting
		Obtain and evaluate ABGs
	Lack of sleep	Check sleep record and provide for sleep
Somnolence, obtundation	Response to drugs, rising Pa_{CO_2}	Check and evaluate medication record; if not easily explained, obtain and evaluate ABGs
Complaints		
Dyspnea	Anxiety	Reassure, alleviate fears
	$\downarrow Pa_{O_2}$	Check patient-ventilator system; if not easily corrected, obtain and evaluate ABGs
	$\downarrow$ Ventilation	
	Pneumothorax	Obtain and evaluate chest x-ray film
Headache	Rising Pa_{CO_2}	Check patient-ventilator system; if not easily explained, obtain and evaluate ABGs
Spontaneous activity		
Twitching, tetany, convulsions	$\downarrow Pa_{CO_2}$ with rising pH	Check patient-ventilator system; if not otherwise explained, obtain and evaluate ABGs
Asterixis	$\uparrow Pa_{CO_2}$	If not otherwise explained, obtain and evaluate ABGs

Table 5 Vital signs

Clue	Possible problem	Advice
Hypotension	↓Venous return (caused by changes in intrathoracic pressure)	Evaluate fluid balance and possible need for filling of vascular bed
Hypertension	Anxiety	Reassure, alleviate fears
	Early response to ↓Pa_{O_2}, ↓Pa_{CO_2}	Check patient-ventilator system; if not easily correctable, obtain and evaluate ABGs
Respiratory swing of blood pressure	↓Venous return (caused by changes in intrathoracic pressure)	If systolic and diastolic pressures below levels for adequate perfusion, evaluate fluid balance and consider filling vascular bed
New arrhythmias, tachycardia, bradycardia	Anxiety	Reassure, alleviate fears
	↓Pa_{O_2}, ↓Pa_{CO_2}, ↑Pa_{CO_2}	Check patient-ventilator system; if not quickly correctable, obtain and evaluate ABGs
	↓Venous return	Check other hemodynamic parameters for adequacy of perfusion
Large swings in CVP or PAW	↓Venous return	Evaluate other hemodynamic parameters for adequacy of perfusion
↓Urinary output	Decreased cardiac output due to decreased venous return	Evaluate other hemodynamic parameters for adequacy of perfusion
Fever	↑Metabolic rate caused by ↑ inspiratory effort or patient-ventilator asynchrony	Check sensitivity and patient triggering effort settings
	Infection	Treat infection; review preventive measures
	Atelectasis	Check patient-ventilator system for secretions, plugs, slippage of tube into right main stem bronchus
	Overheated humidifier	Check temperature setting of humidifier heater
Weight gain	Fluid retention caused by ↓venous return	Evaluate other hemodynamic parameters for adequacy of perfusion; consider diuresis
Changes in respiratory rate	Altered settings	Check patient-ventilator settings
	Change in metabolic needs	Evaluate patient metabolic rate
	Anxiety	Reassure, alleviate fears
	Sleep	Normal—metabolic rate is decreased

Table 6 Physical examination

Clue	Possible problem	Advice
Chest signs		
Asynchrony with the ventilator	Anxiety	Reassure; alleviate fears
	Inadequate flow rate	Check patient-ventilator settings
	Inappropriate I:E ratio	Immediately correct asynchrony by hand-bagging with an $F_{I_{O_2}}$ of 1.0 until cause is identified and corrected
	$\downarrow Pa_{O_2}$, $\uparrow Pa_{CO_2}$	If not easily corrected, obtain and evaluate ABGs
Air leak via chest tube	New pneumothorax	Obtain and evaluate chest x-ray film
	Rupture of blebs	Obtain and evaluate ABGs; alter ventilation as needed
$\downarrow$Breath sounds	Decreased tidal volume	Check patient-ventilator system
	Atelectasis	Check chest x-ray film for position of tube, new lung infiltrates, or pneumothorax
	Pneumonia	
	Tube down right main stem bronchus	
	Pneumothorax	
Rhonchi	Secretions	Clear airway of secretions
	Moisture from tubings draining into trachea	Reposition ventilator tubings
Wheezing	Bronchospasm	Check patient-ventilator system
	High flow rate	
Skin		
Cool skin, diminished pulses	Vasoconstriction resulting from decreased cardiac output	Check other hemodynamic parameters for adequacy of perfusion
	$\downarrow Pa_{CO_2}$, $\downarrow Pa_{O_2}$	Check patient-ventilator system; if not otherwise explained, obtain and evaluate ABGs
Hot moist skin	$\uparrow Pa_{CO_2}$	Check patient-ventilator system; if not otherwise explained, obtain and evaluate ABGs
Subcutaneous emphysema	If tracheostomy present, air may dissect into soft tissues of neck	Reposition and secure tracheostomy tube
	Pneumothorax	Chest x-ray film stat; treat pneumothorax with chest tube
Airway and secretions		
Air leak around endotracheal tube	Inadequate cuff inflation	Reinflate cuff
	Ruptured cuff	Replace endotracheal tube
	Tracheoesophageal fistula	Consult other sources
Thick, inspissated secretions	Inadequate humidity	Increase humidity
Copious thin secretions	Overly generous humidity	Check humidifier settings
	Draining of moisture from tubing into trachea	Reposition ventilator tubings

Continued.

Table 6 Physical examination—cont'd

Clue	Possible problem	Advice
Abdomen		
Gastric distention	Air swallowing	Decompress stomach with nasogastric tube
	Excessive inspiratory effort by patient	Check sensitivity setting

Table 7 Laboratory work and x-ray film

Clue	Possible problem	Advice
Blood gases		
$\downarrow Pa_{CO_2}$	Increased ventilation	Check patient-ventilator system
	Decreased metabolic demand	Evaluate patient's demand
	Anxiety-producing situation	Reassure; alleviate fears
	Metabolic acidosis	Correct metabolic acidosis
$\uparrow Pa_{CO_2}$	Decreased ventilation; leaks via endotracheal or chest tube	Check patient-ventilator system
	Right main stem intubation	Check position of tube
	Secretions; obstruction of airway	Clear airway of secretions
	Oversedation	Check medication record
	Increased metabolic demand	Evaluate patient's demand
$\downarrow Pa_{O_2}$	Disconnections, leaks	Check patient-ventilator system
	Decreased ventilation; altered $F_{I_{O_2}}$	Check settings
	Secretions; obstruction of airway	Clear airway of secretions or obstructions
	Right main stem intubation	Verify position of endotracheal tube
Electrolytes		
Hyperkalemia	Acidosis	Obtain and evaluate ABGs
Hypokalemia	Alkalosis	Obtain and evaluate ABGs
Hyponatremia	Dilutional—due to water retention if venous return is decreased	Evaluate hemodynamic status and adequacy of perfusion; consider diuresis
X-ray evidence of		
Gastric distention	Excessive inspiratory effort by patient	Check sensitivity and flow rate settings; check nasogastric tube patency
	Ileus	Consult other sources
Pneumothorax	High intra-alveolar pressure	Decompress with chest tube
	Rupture of blebs	
Endotracheal tube misplacement	Slippage of tube into right main stem bronchus, placement too high or too low	Reposition and secure tube

CHAPTER 15

Monitoring the ventilator

Goal The goal of monitoring is to detect problems early when they are easier to correct.

Principle The ventilator portion of the patient-ventilator system should be checked in a systematic way at least every 1 to 2 hours. The unstable patient-ventilator system may require continuous monitoring and assessment. The monitoring routine should distinguish between conditions that simply need to be checked ("Are things still ok?") and those that need to be measured and recorded.

Review your routine We recommend that you examine your present method of monitoring the ventilator to ensure that mechanisms for observation and recording are adequate, clearly understood, and followed by all team members.

We have previously recommended that a nurse or a therapist be within sight and sound of every patient being ventilated. This should permit frequent evaluation of ventilator function. A systematic evaluation routine should be established for ventilator patients in your particular intensive care unit. Each team member should learn and use the same routine procedures, which should include a ventilator flow chart that permits recording of routine measurements as well as concurrent blood gas measurements.

Scanning and checking The nurse and the therapist should be able to monitor some aspects of ventilator function continuously. Familiarity with the sounds that the normally functioning ventilator makes is useful in identifying early problems.

Periodically, every hour or two, the therapist or the nurse should direct conscious attention to measurement and evaluation of specific parameters. These parameters should be recorded on a flow sheet that should be kept on or near the ventilator. Each set of data should include the time, initials of the individual making the measurements, and a note of explanation for any changes made in the setting.

Evaluating, measuring, recording	*What to measure*	*How often*

Evaluating, measuring, recording

What to measure

Tidal volume
Respiratory rate
Maximum inspiratory pressure
F_{IO_2}
I : E ratio
Inspired gas temperature
Inspiratory flow rate
Assist or control mode
Dead space volume
Alarm status
Sigh volume
Static pressure (if ordered and in-
  dicated)
PEEP

How often

Every 1 to 2 hours and whenever sus-
picions of malfunctions exist

Check routinely but record simply

The following also should be done routinely at appropriate intervals. We suggest that the recording system be as simple as possible. For example, all such checks could be clustered and acknowledged with a single entry such as a check mark or set of initials.

Tubing checked and seen to be clear of water
Humidifier container refilled
Alarm systems checked
Filters checked or replaced
Leaks controlled
Ventilator circuit replaced

Static pressure

Measuring static pressure requires a special maneuver that is described in detail on p. 51. This measurement is usually not routine. However, it is indicated if maximum inspiratory pressure rises sharply or compliance seems to be fluctuating.

Recording blood gas levels

Although, technically, taking blood gas measurements is part of patient monitoring, it is important to record blood gas levels along with the results of ventilator monitoring. Blood gas levels should be recorded in a way *that indicates which ventilator settings produced those levels.* This is usually accomplished by entering both sets of data in the same row or column of the flow sheet.

Respiratory therapy
ventilator flow chart

	Date												
	Time												
Arterial blood gases	Temp (°C)												
	FI_{O_2}												
	pH												
	P_{CO_2}												
	P_{O_2}												
	% Sat												
	HCO_3^-												
	Base excess												
Mode	Ventilator (type/name)												
	Assist/control												
	Mask Cann T piece M-O-M												
Ventilator settings	Tidal volume												
	Respiratory rate												
	MIP												
	Static pressure												
	PEEP												
	Dead space												
	Sigh												
	FE_{CO_2}												
	IFR												
Spontaneous ventilation	Vital capacity												
	Tidal volume												
	Insp. force												
	Resp. rate												

Laboratory data	Date/time			Date/time			Date/time			
	K^+			Na^+			BUN			
	Cl^-			HCT/HB			Creatinine			

CHAPTER 16

Troubleshooting: clues the ventilator offers

Introduction
When routine monitoring of the ventilator discloses a problem or a potential problem, a search for the cause should begin. Adequate ventilation should be assured by using a manual resuscitation bag, if necessary, while the problem is being investigated. This chapter offers suggestions for identifying and correcting such problems.

Ventilator operation systems
A few situations external to machine functioning can develop and cause malfunction of the patient-ventilator system. Team members should keep these situations in the backs of their minds for times when routine troubleshooting fails to result in discovering the causes of problems.

To deliver supplemental oxygen, all volume ventilators depend on a source of high pressure gas. If the oxygen line fails, the ventilator is unable to deliver the proper concentration of oxygen and, in some instances, the volume that is desired.

Most institutions now have backup generators to provide power during power failures. However, if a hospital is not supplied with emergency power during a brown-out or a power loss, a ventilator may malfunction, or more likely, cease to function altogether.

If a heavy piece of equipment is rolled onto the oxygen hose, the hose may be compressed to a degree sufficient to cause decreased delivery of oxygen.

If fluid of any sort is accidentally spilled into the circuitry of the ventilator, the machine will malfunction or cease to function.

Ventilator electrical cords need to be in good working order to assure appropriate ventilator function. Should a ventilator electrical cord have a nonfunctioning ground wire, sufficient leak may exist in the electrical circuit to cause malfunction of other equipment, such as cardiac monitors.

Ventilator-related problems
Most problems with the ventilator are discussed in the troubleshooting table that follows. However, there will be occasions when the routine monitoring that we suggest will not lead team members to discover the cause of a prob-

lem. It is beyond the scope of this manual to discuss the internal function of each ventilator, but the therapists should be prepared to investigate the "guts" of the ventilator for causes of malfunction.

Check the system and settings
Throughout the troubleshooting table you will often be advised to check the patient-ventilator system. This means double-check the settings, consider the possibility that resets have been made, and look for leaks, obstructions, and other common problems.

Table 8 Troubleshooting the ventilator

Clue	Possible reason	Advice
Decreased minute or tidal volume	Leak around endotracheal tube, from the system, or through the chest tube	Check all connections for leaks
	Decreased patient-triggered respiratory rate	Check respiratory rate
	Decreased lung compliance	Evaluate patient
	Airway secretions	Clear airway of secretions
	Altered settings	Check patient-ventilator system
	Malfunctioning spirometer	Calibrate spirometer
Increased minute or tidal volume	Increased patient-triggered respiratory rate	Check respiratory rate
	Altered settings	Check patient-ventilator system
	Hypoxia	Evaluate patient; consider ABGs
	Increased lung compliance	*Good news*
	Malfunctioning spirometer	Calibrate spirometer
Change in respiratory rate	Altered setting	Check patient-ventilator system
	Increased metabolic demand	Evaluate patient
	Hypoxia	Evaluate patient; consider ABGs
Sudden increase in maximum inspiratory pressure	Coughing	Alleviate uncontrolled coughing
	Airway secretions or plugs	Clear airway secretions
	Ventilator tubing kinked or filled with water	Check for kinks and water
	Kinked endotracheal tube	Check for kinks
	Changes in patient position	Consider repositioning
	Endotracheal tube in right main stem bronchus	Verify position
	Patient-ventilator asynchrony	Correct asynchrony
	Bronchospasm	Identify cause and treat
	Pneumothorax	Decompress chest
Gradual increase in maximum inspiratory pressure	Increased lung stiffness	Measure static pressure
	Diffuse obstructive process	Evaluate for reversible problems: Atelectasis Increased lung water Bronchospasm
Sudden decrease in maximum inspiratory pressure	Volume loss from leaks in system	Check patient-ventilator system for leaks
	Clearing of secretions; relief of bronchospasm; increasing compliance	*Good news*

Table 8 Troubleshooting the ventilator—cont'd

Clue	Possible reason	Advice
F_{IO_2} drift	O_2 analyzer error	Calibrate analyzer
	Blender piping failure	Correct failure
	O_2 source failure	Correct failure
	O_2 reservoir leak	Check ventilator reservoir
I:E ratio exceeding 1:3 or less than 1:1½	Altered inspiratory flow rate	Check IFR setting and correct
	Alteration in other settings without compensating flow rate	Check IFR setting and correct
	Alteration of sensitivity setting	Check and correct
	Airway secretions (pressure ventilator)	Clear airway of secretions
	Subtle leaks	Measure minute ventilation
Inspired gas temperature inappropriate	Addition of cool water to humidifier	Wait
	Altered settings	Correct temperature control setting
	Thermostat failure	Replace heater
Changes in delivered PEEP	If ventilator control used: Changes in compliance Changes in tidal volume	Correct problem if possible; if not, increase PEEP setting to to deliver desired level of PEEP
	If external PEEP source used: Evaporation of water Disconnection of expiratory tubing from PEEP device	Add water; check and reconnect
Changes in static pressure	Changes in lung compliance	Evaluate patient and correct cause if possible
Changes in inspiratory flow rate, sigh volume, assist or control mode, alarm status, dead space volume	Changes in these settings result from deliberate or accidental adjustment of dials or knobs	Check to determine whether current settings are accidental or deliberate

CHAPTER 17

Patient comfort

Introduction Patients in respiratory distress often experience a great sense of relief when they first receive assisted or controlled ventilation. The patient is relieved to be free of dyspnea and is content to relax in spite of being tethered by an endotracheal tube. Later, when these patients have settled down, they may become aware of some discomfort. Often, the problems causing such discomfort can be corrected. In this chapter, some causes of patient discomfort are discussed, and possible solutions are suggested.

Goals Easy, comfortable ventilation of the patient in synchrony with the ventilator
Maximum psychological comfort

Physical discomfort Listed for your consideration are some common causes of discomfort experienced by the patient being ventilated.
  Discomfort unrelated to the ventilator
    Real pain
    Awkward positions
    Distended hollow organs
  Discomfort related to the ventilator
    Ability to take only shallow breaths
    Hypoxia
    Heavy tubing
    Loss of ability to speak
    Fear of falling
    Impaired ability to cough
    Inability to yawn or sigh
    Inadequate oral hygiene
    Impaired ability to swallow
    Inactivity and deconditioning
    Overheated air

Psychological discomfort The patient attached to a ventilator loses autonomy over a critical life function—breathing. In addition, he often loses control of other aspects of his physical and psychological self. We list some common causes of psychological discomfort.

Failure of the practitioner to explain procedures
Inadequate information about
    Why ventilation is needed
    Reliability of machine function
    Presence, purpose, and sound of alarms
    Purposes of activities of the team
    Skill of the practitioners
Inability to summon help
Lack of privacy
Loss of control over physical mobility
Loss of sleep
Sensory deprivation or overstimulation
Loss of power and control
Sense of being an object

Physical discomfort

Discomfort unrelated to ventilator
Recognize that some causes of physical discomfort are unrelated to mechanical ventilation, and treat appropriately.

Pain
The patient may be in pain. Pain from surgical incisions, myocardial infarction, or other sources should be alleviated. Small doses of intravenous narcotics titrated to effect are recommended. For example, 2 mg of morphine sulfate (up to 8 mg over 4 hours) seldom causes problems. However, in some patients sympathetic tone may be reduced, and, especially in hypovolemic patients, blood pressure may fall. Fluid replacement usually corrects this drop.

Awkward positions
Awkward or monotonous positions may cause sufficient discomfort to produce patient asynchrony with the ventilator. Frequent position changes are desirable for comfort. In addition to increasing comfort, turning the patient every 1 to 2 hours facilitates better distribution of ventilation and perfusion, promotes circulation, prevents the formation of pressure areas, and provides the stimulus and comfort of touch.

If positioned in good alignment, most patients do not require propping with pillows, but some require pillows behind their backs or between bony prominences of the legs. Most noncardiac patients are comfortable in a supine position with the knees slightly flexed. Cardiac patients often prefer to have the head of the bed elevated 30 degrees or more.

Distended hollow organs
Distended hollow organs, such as bladder, stomach, or intestine, may cause serious discomfort. Decompress appropriately, and avoid actions that will cause redistention.

Discomfort related to ventilator
The patient may have physical discomfort or loss of function because of mechanical ventilation. Some of these are discussed below.

Ability to take only shallow breaths
Improper adjustment of the ventilator settings may lead to discomfort and distress. A common cause of patient discomfort and anxiety is a tidal volume that is too small. Slow, deep breaths are usually much more satisfying than rapid, shallow breaths. If you suspect that tidal volume is too small, check whether the same minute volume can be safely achieved (MIP less than 50) with larger tidal volumes (VT up to 15 ml/kg). If volume and rate settings are inadequate to meet the patient's metabolic needs, severe distress and physiologic impairment may result.

Hypoxia
Inadequate delivery of oxygen to the tissues may cause physical distress. Whenever there is any doubt about the cause of restlessness, confusion, tachycardia, or change in blood pressure, draw a blood gas sample, and *immediately* raise the $F_{I_{O_2}}$. It is highly undesirable to administer narcotics or

hypnotics to a patient whose level of oxygenation is in question. *Always* verify adequacy of oxygenation before administering drugs. Correction of hypoxemia is discussed elsewhere in this book.

Heavy tubing   The weight of the ventilator tubing may cause pulling and tugging on the mouth, nares, or throat. This causes pain as well as injury to tissues. Securing the endotracheal tube to the face with tape should be done in a way that protects the tissues yet assures stability. Discomfort can be decreased by properly positioning and supporting the tubing and using flexible connectors to keep weight off the facial structures.

Loss of ability to speak   Inability to speak causes distress for most patients. The patient should be reassured that the ability to speak will return as soon as the tube is removed. Alternate methods of communication, including lipreading, magic slates, paper and pencil, alphabet boards, and lists of common needs and questions, should be used. Fear can result from the inability to call out for help. Even through a nurse is constantly present, the patient should have a means of attracting attention. Signal lights, bells, or something with which to bang the siderails should be easily available to the patient.

Fear of falling   Most patients attached to ventilators have their beds in the high position for ease of care. There is a real and constant danger that inadvertent movement of the patient may lead to a fall from the bed. The siderails should *always* be in the raised position, even though a nurse is always present.

Impaired ability to cough   The ability to cough is decreased during mechanical ventilation because of the inability to close the glottis. The large airways should be kept clear by suctioning. The small airways and alveoli should be cleared by appropriate humidification, percussion, vibration, and postural drainage. Accumulation of secretions or saliva may be cleared from the back of the throat or mouth with a tonsil tip sucker. Encourage the patient to cough actively before and during suctioning to facilitate removal of deep secretions and to maintain the strength of breathing and coughing muscles.

Inability to yawn or sigh   Loss of the normal sigh mechanism (yawning) should be replaced by setting the ventilator sigh or by manually hyperinflating the patient for several breaths every 5 to 10 minutes. Ventilating with a bag is a good way to do this, since rate and depth can be varied easily.

Inadequate oral hygiene   Mouth care is especially important for the patient who has an artificial airway. Frequent repositioning of an orotracheal tube from one side of the mouth to the other will help prevent buccal irritation and possible ulceration.

Impaired ability to swallow   The patient may have difficulty in swallowing. Excess secretions and saliva can cause discomfort or become a source of infection, or they may be aspirated. A tonsil tip sucker can be used to make oral suctioning as atraumatic as possible. If the oral secretions are copious, the patient should be taught to handle the tonsil tip sucker.

Some intubated patients tend to swallow air. A nasogastric tube should be inserted to prevent gastric distention and possible regurgitation and aspiration. If the patient is alert and swallowing seems normal, this tube may be removed after decompression. However, the degree of gastric distention should be assessed frequently. If a nasogastric tube is required for days or weeks, a soft silicone rubber tube should be used.

If the patient is receiving oral or nasogastric feedings, his head should be elevated during feedings and for about 30 minutes after feedings. Obviously, the cuff should also be inflated during this time.

Inactivity and deconditioning   Connection of a patient to a mechanical ventilator often leads to decreased activity that causes loss of skeletal and respiratory muscle mass. To minimize respiratory muscle loss, the patient should be triggering the ventilator whenever possible, and breathing exercises should be done. To minimize skeletal muscle loss and decrease of strength, assistive and active joint range-of-motion exercises should be done every few hours as soon as a steady state is reached. If the patient is to be ventilated more than 24 hours and is stable hemodynamically, consider having him sit in a chair or walk about the bedside or down the halls, as described on pp. 103 and 104.

Postural hypotension may occur. Therefore, each level of mobilization should be carefully monitored by observing heart rate and blood pressure.

Reassurance should be given to the patient regarding the safety and desirability of such activity. Adequate personnel should be on hand to prevent problems as well as to reassure the patient that plenty of help is available.

Dependence on the ventilator may develop for physical (for example, ventilatory muscle mass loss) and psychological reasons. Once his condition is stabilized, the patient should be reassured that mechanical ventilation is temporary and that normal breathing will resume as his condition improves.

Physical restraints limit active movement and should be used *only* in the unlikely event that the patient traumatizes his airway by pulling or tugging on the endotracheal tube.

Overheated air   The temperature of the inspired gas should be maintained approximately at body temperature. This may cause some patients to feel very uncomfortable. Explanation and a slight decrease in this temperature may be helpful.

Psychological discomfort

General   The patient being mechanically ventilated loses autonomy over a vital body function—breathing. In addition, because he is often critically ill, he loses autonomy over most activities. He is expected to trustingly permit others to manipulate his physical and psychological self, his environment, and his significant others. A formerly independent, self-reliant human being must breath artificially and be fed intravenously; he is dressed and undressed, bathed, pulled, pushed, and moved about without much control over his keepers or himself. Finally, he finds his physical and psychological nakedness exposed to strangers who have varying levels of empathy.

The cost of coping Despite limited levels of energy, the patient must direct some energy toward coping with psychological stress. We can, by being aware of and responsive to his psychological needs, minimize the energy required for such coping.

Families can compound the problem by expecting higher levels of interaction from the patient than he is capable of giving. Carefully including the family or significant others in explanations and in the care of the patient is much more desirable than the creation of artificial "visiting hours."

Psychological discomfort caused by ventilator Many aspects of the psychological stress that the patient undergoes are directly related to ventilator management and function.

Failure to explain It is important to remember that what is familiar and safe for us may be a new and terrifying experience for the patient. On each approach to the patient, you should tell him what you are looking for or doing and what you expect to find and give him a reasonable explanation for what is found unless such facts are recognizably repetitive *to the patient*. New information given to the patient should *correctly* add to, make current, confirm, and be consistent with information he has already been given.

Information the patient often wants Information given to the patient should, of course, be accurate and should be given in a manner that does not create anxiety. A calm, matter-of-fact approach is reassuring. Many patients have expressed questions about the following:

> Why ventilation is needed
> Reliability of machine function (whether it will "turn on" and "turn off" as often as they need breaths)
> Whether alarms exist
> What alarms mean when they sound
> Purposes of the activities of personnel around them (routine checking, testing, filling of humidifiers)
> Skill of the personnel

Many other questions arise, and they should be answered.

Knowing how to get help We highly recommend that a nurse stay within sight of a patient being ventilated, not only for maintenance of the system but also for the psychological comfort of the patient. Should the nurse need to leave the immediate area of the patient, another professional should be in attendance. Even though a nurse or a therapist is present, the patient should have a means to attract attention.

Lack of privacy Our insistence on the presence of a qualified person at the bedside denies privacy to the patient. Privacy is needed for personal autonomy, emotional release, self integration, and protected communication. It is helpful to remember that "initimate" territory is considered to be within 18 inches, "personal" distance 18 inches to 3 feet, and "social" distance 3 to 13 feet. Constant intrusion into personal space by many people can cause stress, fatigue, or fear. Activities should therefore be organized to keep personnel at a "social" distance whenever immediate actions are not required.

Every precaution should be taken to prevent phsycial exposure of the patient to other patients and visitors—indeed, to anyone other than those with a "need to know."

Loss of control over physical mobility In addition to the many physiologic reasons for mobility, the psychological aspect is important. A patient's sense of powerlessness can be decreased by allowing him maximal control over such normal activities as turning, getting up in a chair, or taking care of his own body. His attitude toward recovery improves as he regains control of motions.

Loss of sleep Although not completely understood, the need for sleep in the maintenance of healthy psyche and soma is well recognized. When the patient's condition has become stable, the team must carefully organize activities and monitoring around planned sleep or rest periods to decrease the psychological insult to the patient. Safe monitoring of the patient-ventilator system may be carried out while the patient is sleeping, particularly if an arterial line is in place for blood pressure readings.

Sensory deprivation The team should minimize unfamiliar noises, create a familiar environment, explain support devices, and allow the patient to have some possessions. Wearing name tags, introducing yourself and other team members, describing the physical setting, and having clocks and calendars in view help to orient the patient to his environment.

Disorientation may also result from overloading the patient's sensory system. As discussed previously, sleep and privacy are important.

Loss of significant social interaction The patient can experience excruciating loneliness and despair, a sense of meaninglessness, and shattering feelings of impotency caused by isolation from friends and family. Significant others should be allowed to continue to support the patient's fragile image as a loved one. If family members or friends are not present, nurses, therapists, and physicians must provide interactions that go beyond the patient as a sick person.

Loss of power and control The patient may feel a loss of power and control over his body as well as his environment. When possible, the patient should be a part of the creation of his own "future," even if the future is the next hour. If not energy depleting, decisions regarding times for baths, meals, activities, visitors, and therapeutic maneuvers should be made by the patient. Changes of bed location within the ICU should be explained carefully to prevent feelings of isolation or punishment.

Sense of being an object There is an unfortunate tendency to talk about the patient as an object or a problem (for example, "the mitral valve in Room 6"). At the bedside this attitude is reflected in the tendency to speak about the patient as if he could not hear.

Whenever possible, use the patient's name. At the bedside of a patient who is alert, acknowledge his presence in the same way you speak to others in the room.

Summary We are learning more and more about the areas of physical and psychological concern to the patient undergoing continuous ventilation. Although overworked, the request "Treat me like a human being" applies to the care these patients deserve. A thoughtful, empathic approach usually takes care of most of the physical and psychological insults to which these patients are subjected. Such thoughtfulness and empathy may require a conscious effort at first.

A caution There is real danger that the psychological care given to the patient will be based not on the *patient's* needs but rather on the *practitioner's* needs or perceptions. What the practitioner has "read" or found appropriate for one patient, or senses is the "right thing to do," may not be right for another patient.

When assessing psychological needs of the patient as a basis for planning professional intervention, the entire team should be involved to minimize misconceptions by individual team members. If the problems, either of the patient or of the staff, seem insurmountable, a consultation from a psychiatric nurse or physician may be useful in determining a consistent approach.

A patient care plan should be *written* and followed by the entire team. The patient should not be expected to change his methods of coping when dealing with different team members.

CHAPTER 18

Bagging

Introduction Other chapters of this book make reference to "bagging." This means using a resuscitation bag to ventilate a patient. We will now describe bagging in some detail.

A bag for each patient It is recommended that a resuscitation bag be available at the bedside of each patient undergoing mechanical ventilation.

When to bag Bagging is a technique used when the:
Ventilator fails
Patient is suctioned
Patient is ambulated
Patient is dyspneic and/or "out of phase"
Ventilator must be disconnected to be serviced or checked

Ventilator failure If the ventilator or its power source fails, an alternative method of ventilating the patient must be available immediately. For this reason alone, a resuscitation bag and a trained person should be available at the patient's bedside at all times.

Suctioning When a patient is suctioned for secretions, air is also removed from the lungs. The effects of this removal of air can be reduced by hyperinflating and hyperoxygenating the patient before and after suctioning. Although it is possible to hyperinflate and hyperoxygenate by changing the ventilator settings, it is usually easier to use a resuscitation bag.

Resetting the ventilator to hyperoxygenate and hyperinflate when the patient is suctioned has two disadvantages. First, the reset ventilator is limited to one tidal volume or respiratory rate, whereas changes in volume and rate are easily arranged with a bag. Second, if the ventilator is reset to hyperinflate and oxygenate, the controls need to be corrected to their original settings, and a busy staff may forget to do so. This may lead to inappropriately high $F_{I_{O_2}}$s or volumes.

Ambulating patients It is cumbersome to try to ambulate a patient tethered to a ventilator. When a patient is to be ambulated, it is easier to ventilate him with a bag and small oxygen tank. Because it is easier, the patient and staff are more likely to attempt ambulation earlier. This enhances reconditioning and makes weaning easier.

Dyspneic and "out of phase" Patients are often dyspneic and asynchronous, or "out of phase," when they are first connected to the ventilator. Patients who seem well adjusted to the ventilator may also become dyspneic or "out of phase" for various other reasons.

If the patient is asynchronous with the ventilator or is dyspneic, additional ventilation and oxygenation can easily be provided with a bag. Rapid breaths can be provided to alleviate the feeling of dyspnea or to "blow off" CO_2 to regain synchrony with mechanical ventilation. As control and relaxation are achieved, the breaths easily can be made slower and deeper.

If a patient is short of breath, whether from a physiologic cause or because of anxiety, he should be provided with additional ventilation immediately. It is of no value whatever to tell the patient to slow his breathing or to breathe more deeply when he is acutely anxious. The patient should be ventilated with a high $F_{I_{O_2}}$ (unless absolute contraindication exists) until the perceived and real needs of the patient are met.

When initiating such ventilation, you should ventilate "with the patient," that is, at his rate, but at a deeper volume. As the deeper volume that you are delivering "satisfies" the patient, the rate may be slowed. At no time should the nurse or the therapist ventilate asynchronously with the patient. If the patient's respiratory rate is too rapid to permit bagging with deep breaths, control may be regained by bagging even more rapidly than the patient is breathing. When control is regained, the depth of the breath can be increased and the rate slowed.

It is useful to have one or two lengths (6 to 12 inches) of dead-space tubing attached to the head of the bag. This extra tubing allows the therapist or the nurse to bag more easily (with one hand if necessary) and the bag to be held out of the patient's sight. This tends to reduce anxiety.

Resuscitation bags—good and bad

Selection There are many brands of resuscitation bags on the market. Selection of a bag should be based on a number of factors which we will now address.

Characteristics of a good system There are basically five areas of function that should be considered in selecting a good resuscitation bag system. They are:

1. Ventilation
2. Oxygenation
3. Modification for use with PEEP equipment
4. Operation
5. Cleaning

Ventilation A good system should be capable of delivering a minimum of 1000 ml tidal volume. The bag should refill quickly to assure ability to deliver rapid tidal breaths of this volume. The bag should be easy to manipulate by persons with various sizes of hands.

Oxygenation A good system should come equipped with a fitting that accepts oxygen via small-bore tubing. When connected to a high flow of oxygen, the system will deliver various concentrations of oxygen depending on the type of bag used.

A good system also should be equipped with a fitting that accepts wide-bore tubing to be used as a reservoir. This reservoir should increase the $F_{I_{O_2}}$ capability to 0.7. Some systems come equipped with the capability to deliver 0.7 or higher concentrations without a reservoir tail.

It should be possible to adapt the system to deliver an $F_{I_{O_2}}$ of 1.0. In some systems an adapter is available from the manufacturer. In other systems an adapter must be improvised. For example, an $F_{I_{O_2}}$ of 1.0 can be obtained with assurance if a large-volume reservoir (10 to 100 L) is attached to the intake port of the bag and connected directly to an oxygen source.

PEEP A good system will allow for easy modification for use with PEEP. PEEP equipment can be attached to most bag exhalation valves by using either ball valves or wide-bore tubing between the exhalation valve and a water column PEEP device.

Many modifications of bagging systems to obtain 100% O_2 and to maintain PEEP have been supported recently in respiratory therapy journals.

Bags that have "fish mouth" valves do not lend themselves easily to adaptation for PEEP.

Operation of the system A good resuscitation bagging system is constructed to prevent clogging of the inflation valve should the patient have copious secretions. It permits the patient to operate this valve without the necessity of manual compression of the bag. A good system also allows for the use of high oxygen flow rates while eliminating the possibility of the inflation valve becoming jammed in the "inflate" position.

Cleaning and assembly

A good system allows for sterilization and cleaning. Bags that have foam rubber interiors are not recommended because they cannot be washed on the interior and should not be gas autoclaved.

A good system also employs color coding of ports to minimize the possibility of improper assembly.

CHAPTER 19

Suctioning the airway

Introduction Suctioning the airway is an essential part of the care of the patient who has an endotracheal tube, which interferes with closure of the glottis and precludes effective, "explosive" coughing.

Principle Secretions in the larger airways must be removed by suctioning. The suction catheter will reach only the first division of the major bronchi. Secretions must be moved to these larger airways by coughing, postural drainage, percussion, and vibration. These measures should precede suctioning.

Goal The goal of endotracheal suctioning is to remove secretions from the upper airway.

Basic rule This procedure should be carried out *only* on indication. "Routine" hourly suctioning is damaging to the trachea and painful to the patient, and involves serious risk. "Routine" suctioning is, therefore, to be avoided.

Indication The *only* indication for suctioning is the presence of secretions in the upper airway. Such secretions are detected by auscultation.

Precautions It is important to take certain precautions when you suction a patient:
Oxygenate immediately before and after suctioning.
Avoid prolonged suctioning (more than 10 seconds at a time).
Monitor the ECG for arrhythmias throughout the suctioning procedure.

Suctioning procedure The following procedure is recommended for ventilator patients:
1. Auscultate the chest to verify the presence of rhonchi in large airways.
2. Assemble the equipment:
   a. Sterile catheter and glove
   b. Suction source at medium (120 mm/Hg or less) setting
   c. Resuscitator bag attached to oxygen source or—ventilator set at an FI_{O_2} of 1.0
   d. 3 ml syringe filled with normal saline solution
   e. Water or normal saline solution for catheter rinse
3. Describe the procedure to the patient.

4. Mobilize the secretions in the smaller airways with chest physical therapy.
5. Observe the ECG monitor throughout the procedure.
6. Preoxygenate and hyperinflate with a resuscitator bag or the manual control on the ventilator for 30 seconds or 6 to 8 breaths.
7. Insert the catheter and advance it quickly until resistance is met. Do not apply suction while advancing, and do not force the catheter.
8. Pull the catheter back 1 cm, then apply suction. Rotate the catheter while withdrawing it. *Apply suction for no more than 10 seconds.*
9. Hyperoxygenate and hyperinflate between each suctioning maneuver and after the final suctioning attempt.
10. If secretions are thick, install normal saline solution, hyperinflate for 3 to 4 breaths, and then suction.
11. Rinse the catheter only after suctioning is completed.
12. If required, suction the patient's nose or mouth after suctioning the trachea.
13. Discard the equipment by wrapping the catheter inside the glove.
14. Auscultate the chest to evaluate the clearing of secretions.
15. Chart the following:
    a. Color, amount, and character of secretions
    b. Patient tolerance
    c. Auscultatory findings
    d. Any complications that occurred

More on suctioning

Selection of suction kits

A number of disposable suctioning kits are commercially available. Such kits are highly recommended for the assurance of sterility and convenience.

When selecting a kit, you should carefully examine its contents. It should be guaranteed sterile. The kit should contain a suction catheter, which should be available in a variety of sizes, a glove, and a rinse cup. The catheter should be soft and pliable and at least 18 inches long, and it should hang straight when removed from the package. The catheter must be equipped with a thumb vent to control suction application.

Complications of suctioning

Improperly performed suctioning can be dangerous. Listed below are some complications that may be encountered when improper technique is used:

Hypoxia—usually caused by prolonged suctioning or inadequate oxygenation prior to suctioning

Dysrhythmias; cardiovascular collapse or cardiac arrest—usually caused by hypoxia or vagal stimulation

Atelectasis—usually caused by subatmospheric intrapulmonic pressures or wedging of the suction catheter in a small bronchus

Trauma

Aspiration

Cross infection

How to avoid complications

Complications can be avoided or minimized by using a careful, consistent technique and by carefully monitoring the cardiac rhythm during the procedure. The three main precautions to take are:

1. Preoxygenate and postoxygenate.
2. Suction no longer than 10 seconds at a time.
3. Monitor cardiac rhythm during the procedure.

Tips on technique

Suctioning is one of the most unpleasant experiences that a ventilator patient has. A thorough explanation and a careful and gentle technique, as well as suctioning only on indication, should minimize the discomfort.

The catheter should not be larger than half the diameter of the endotracheal tube through which it must pass. This decreases the possibility that the catheter will become wedged in the endotracheal tube and cause atelectasis and also minimizes the degree of shortness of breath.

Handwashing with a disinfectant soap before and after suctioning is absolutely essential to prevent cross infection. The use of sterile technique is mandatory.

Suctioning should be preceded by adequate wetting of the secretions for ease of removal. Secretions should then be moved to the upper airway by chest physical therapy maneuvers, such as postural drainage, percussion, and vibration.

The cuff of the endotracheal tube should remain inflated during suctioning to minimize the risk of aspiration if the patient should regurgitate stomach contents.

CHAPTER 20

Physical therapy maneuvers

Introduction   Most patients who are intubated and mechanically ventilated are partially or completely immobilized or have increased chest secretions. Physical therapy maneuvers will enhance movement of joints, muscles, blood, air, and secretions. If such maneuvers have not been part of the patient's treatment, we strongly urge that they be included.

Factors favoring deconditioning   The patient may be too sick or obtunded or in too much pain to exert himself adequately to maintain normal movement. Professionals, in their zealous concern for endotracheal tubes, monitoring lines, intravenous catheters, fractures, or incisions, may discourage the patient from moving about even if he tries. Thus the patient may be relatively inactive for a prolonged period of time if the team neglects exercising joints and muscles.

Bed rest alone deconditions peripheral skeletal muscles within a matter of 1 to 3 days. Therefore, the patient should be kept active and moving. The goal is to decrease the period of convalescence that may be caused by deconditioning.

Skeletal muscle   Skeletal muscles atrophy with disuse. A patient's range of motion may be limited because he is tethered to lines and tubes. In addition, the cardiovascular system begins adapting to an exertion-free existence and decreases its functioning level. Venous return is no longer augmented by the activity of skeletal muscle.

Joints   Joints stiffen rapidly and further inhibit muscular movement.

Respiratory musculature   The patient undergoing mechanical ventilation may have limited drive or need to breathe on his own. The muscles of respiration (chiefly the diaphragm) become weak from disuse. The patient's voluntary control over his breathing muscles decreases, making it difficult for him to take segmental and deep breaths voluntarily. This leads to a prolonged weaning period and/ or respiratory problems after extubation.

Suggested routine   We therefore recommend exercises to enhance movement of muscles, joints, blood, air and secretions.

Breathing exercises The patient being artificially ventilated should begin breathing exercises long before weaning—ideally, as soon after intubation as the patient is relaxed, alert, and cooperative.

Goals The goals of breathing exercises in this setting are to maintain the strength of ventilatory muscles and to retain voluntary control of breathing.

Steps 1. Explain the rationale of the exercises.
2. Place gentle pressure with your hand over alternate areas of the chest (left and right lateral rib cage and right and left diaphragms).
3. Tell the patient to push against your hand or to try to move his rib cage out during the inspiratory phase of each ventilator-delivered breath.
4. Tell the patient to follow this "active" inspiration with passive exhalation.

Schedule Frequency of the exercises should be every 2 to 4 hours during waking hours, once the patient's condition is stable. Using the technique described above, facilitate expansion for 4 sigh volume breaths, then for 2 minutes of tidal volume breaths, then for 4 sigh volume breaths.

Rest.

Repeat for each of the four chest areas.

Resistive diaphragmatic breathing Long-term ventilator patients should do resistive diaphragmatic breathing exercises.

Goals The goal of this exercise is to strengthen the diaphragm.

Steps 1. Place the patient in a supine position.
2. Flex the knees.
3. Place a 3 lb sandbag on the abdomen.
4. Instruct the patient to breathe with his diaphragm and raise the sandbag during inspiration.

Schedule Repeat for 3 to 50 breaths as tolerated, 4 times daily.

Active movement Active or active-assistive exercises should be attempted if hemodynamic status permits.

Goals These exercises will promote near-normal joint range of motion (JROM), good muscle tone, and proper function of the vascular system.

Exercises can be done in the supine, semi-Fowler, or sitting position. The head of the bed should be slowly raised while blood pressure and heart rate are monitored to check for postural hypotension. After activity is initiated, the pulse rate should be monitored carefully and frequently to evaluate the level of fatigue. The patient should be positioned comfortably for each exercise.

Steps
1. Shoulder flexion exercises
2. Shoulder horizontal abduction exercises
3. Knee-to-chest exercises
4. Straight leg raises
5. "Bedpans" (knees flexed, feet flat on bed, raise hips as if getting onto a bedpan)
6. Pull-ups and sit-ups with overhead trapeze if available
7. Ankle circles
8. Ambulation

Schedule
Five to ten repetitions of the joint range of motion exercises two to four times daily is recommended. Ankle circles can be done independently by most patients after they are taught. Ten to fifty repetitions hourly while awake are recommended. Be sure the patient has no restriction of ankle motion during these exercises.

Ambulation should begin as soon as the patient is able to tolerate it. Using a walker, a resuscitation bag, portable oxygen, and adequate professional help, even a very sick ventilator patient can walk 2 or 3 times daily.

Passive joint range of motion
Passive JROM exercises should be done only if the patient is comatose or if there is a medical or surgical contraindication to active movement. If no contractures or excess stretch exists in the muscles, daily or twice-daily passive JROM exercises should be adequate.

Percussion
Lung segments with secretions should be clapped with cupped hands. This will greatly aid in the movement of secretions to larger airways. It is vital to position the patient appropriately for each lung area. Be cautious around chest tubes, fractured ribs, and surgical sites.

Goal
The goal of percussion is to faciliate the movement of secretions from alveoli and small airways to larger airways from which they may be coughed up or suctioned.

Steps
1. Determine the frequency of treatments.
2. Explain the procedure to patient.
3. Position the patient appropriately for the lung segment to be percussed.
4. With cupped hands, percuss each affected segment for 2 to 3 minutes or longer.
5. While vibrating the segment, ask the patient to cough on exhalation.
6. If the secretions are not removed by coughing, the patient should be suctioned.
7. Leave the patient in the drainage position for at least 15 minutes.

Schedule
Frequency of treatment should be determined by the quantity of secretions as well as the ability of the patient to tolerate the procedure. Most patients can tolerate the treatment of one lung segment or area after each position

change (every hour or two). Some patients can tolerate having several segments treated sequentially.

Vibration Vibration is a gentler form of "chest shaking" than percussion. Vibration is useful in all patients, but particularly in those with fragile bone structures, those in hyperexpanded states, or those in pain from surgical incisions, trauma, or insertion of tubes.

Goal The goal of vibration is to facilitate the movement of secretions from alveoli and small airways to larger airways from which they may be coughed up or suctioned.

Steps
1. Determine the frequency of treatments.
2. Explain the procedure to the patient.
3. Position the patient. Unlike percussion, vibration may be done in any position.
4. Vibrate the chest by placing your hands one on top of the other, then on the patient's chest, while tensing your forearm muscles sufficiently to cause a fine tremor in your hands. This tremor will produce a vibration in the lung segments under your hands.
5. Vibrate *only* during exhalation.
6. After vibration, have the patient cough. If the secretions are not removed but are in the upper airways, suction.

Schedule Vibration, which is often done in conjunction with percussion, is a useful technique, particularly for patients who are air hungry and must sit upright to breathe. Vibration may be done in any position because it is an expiratory maneuver.

Postural drainage Placing the patient in a postural drainage position will engage gravity to move secretions. Appropriate positioning should be used for each lung segment or area.

Goal The goal of postural drainage is to facilitate the movement of secretions from alveoli and smaller airways to larger airways from which they may be coughed up or suctioned.

Steps
1. Determine which lung segments are affected and require drainage.
2. Select the appropriate drainage position for the area.
3. Explain the procedure to the patient, and position the patient.
4. Observe carefully for any untoward symptoms.
5. If none occur, leave the patient in the position for at least 15 minutes.
6. Repeat the procedure for each segment requiring drainage.

Schedule Frequency of drainage should be determined by the quantity of secretions as well as the ability of the patient to tolerate the procedure. Most patients can tolerate the treatment of one lung segment or area after each position change (every hour or two). Some patients can tolerate having several segments treated sequentially.

The role of the physical therapist If the patient is particularly sick or the team has not treated a ventilator patient recently, managing the patient-ventilator system hour by hour may completely consume the attention of the physician, the nurse, and the respiratory therapist. If the physical therapist is not routinely a part of this team, as is sometimes the case, it may be useful to ask him or her to assist in some or all of these maneuvers.

CHAPTER 21

Positive end-expiratory pressure (PEEP)

Introduction It is difficult to oxygenate some patients in severe respiratory distress without using very high concentrations of oxygen. Some of these patients can be helped by PEEP therapy. However, both the use of PEEP and the administration of high concentrations of oxygen involve risks.

"Best PEEP" For each patient there is a PEEP setting that represents the best compromise between the advantages and disadvantages of PEEP. This level of PEEP is known as "best PEEP." It varies from patient to patient.

The PEEP study The optimum PEEP setting should be determined by a study of each patient's unique responses to various levels of PEEP.

PEEP is used to increase Pa_{O_2}. The effect of PEEP on Pa_{O_2} may be exaggerated by high FI_{O_2}s (see Fig. 6). This means that it may be easier to recognize the "best PEEP" if Pa_{O_2} is measured at different PEEP settings *while the patient is breathing 100% oxygen*. When the optimal PEEP setting is determined, the FI_{O_2} can be reduced as tolerated.

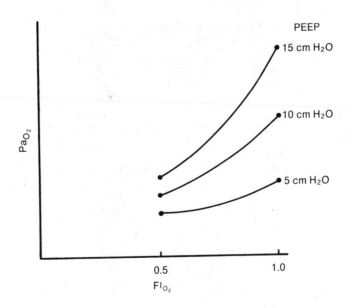

The PEEP study is undertaken with the expectation of testing several different PEEP settings. However, as PEEP is increased in steps, it may become apparent that PEEP settings above a certain level are not well tolerated. When this is recognized, the PEEP study should be terminated. In such a situation, the "best PEEP" should be determined by analysis of the data available from the limited study.

A PEEP study "flow sheet" and algorithm are provided.

PEEP study: flow sheet

Date _____

PEEP (cm H_2O)		0	5	10	15	0
Time started						
MIP (cm H_2O)						
Static pressure						
V_T (liters)						
Systolic	insp.					
(respiratory swing)	exp.					
A-VD_{O_2} (ml O_2/100 ml blood)						
Pa_{O_2}*						
Pa_{CO_2}						

*Assume $F_{I_{O_2}}$ of 1.0.

The PEEP algorithm
Indications and guide to initial settings for patients being ventilated

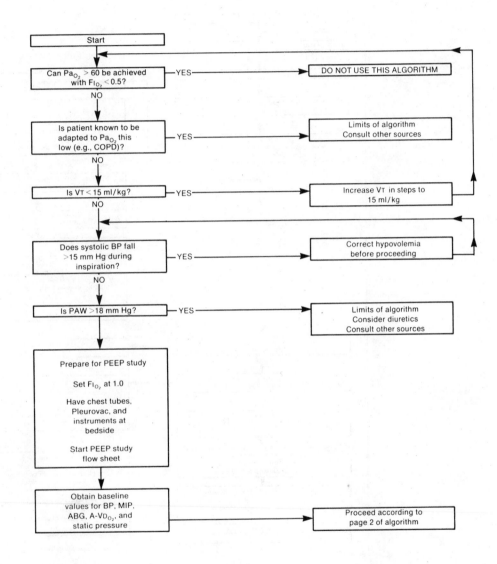

Start

Can $Pa_{O_2} > 60$ be achieved with $F_{I_{O_2}} < 0.5$? —YES— DO NOT USE THIS ALGORITHM

NO

Is patient known to be adapted to Pa_{O_2} this low (e.g., COPD)? —YES— Limits of algorithm / Consult other sources

NO

Is $V_T < 15$ ml/kg? —YES— Increase V_T in steps to 15 ml/kg

NO

Does systolic BP fall >15 mm Hg during inspiration? —YES— Correct hypovolemia before proceeding

NO

Is PAW >18 mm Hg? —YES— Limits of algorithm / Consider diuretics / Consult other sources

Prepare for PEEP study

Set $F_{I_{O_2}}$ at 1.0

Have chest tubes, Pleurovac, and instruments at bedside

Start PEEP study flow sheet

Obtain baseline values for BP, MIP, ABG, $A-V_{D_{O_2}}$, and static pressure → Proceed according to page 2 of algorithm

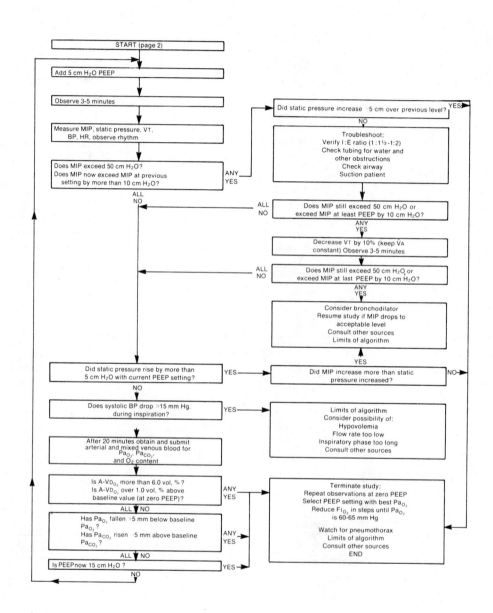

START (page 2)

Add 5 cm H_2O PEEP

Observe 3-5 minutes

Measure MIP, static pressure, V_T,
BP, HR, observe rhythm

Does MIP exceed 50 cm H_2O?
Does MIP now exceed MIP at previous
setting by more than 10 cm H_2O?

ALL NO

Did static pressure increase 5 cm over previous level?

NO

Troubleshoot:
Verify I:E ratio (1:1½-1:2)
Check tubing for water and
other obstructions
Check airway
Suction patient

ANY YES

Does MIP still exceed 50 cm H_2O or
exceed MIP at least PEEP by 10 cm H_2O?

ALL NO

ANY YES

Decrease V_T by 10% (keep V_A
constant) Observe 3-5 minutes

Does MIP still exceed 50 cm H_2O or
exceed MIP at last PEEP by 10 cm H_2O?

ALL NO

ANY YES

Consider bronchodilator
Resume study if MIP drops to
acceptable level
Consult other sources
Limits of algorithm

YES

Did static pressure rise by more than
5 cm H_2O with current PEEP setting?

YES

Did MIP increase more than static
pressure increased?

NO

NO

Does systolic BP drop >15 mm Hg.
during inspiration?

YES

Limits of algorithm
Consider possibility of:
Hypovolemia
Flow rate too low
Inspiratory phase too long
Consult other sources

After 20 minutes obtain and submit
arterial and mixed venous blood for
Pa_{O_2}, Pa_{CO_2},
and O_2 content

Is A-VD_{O_2} more than 6.0 vol, % ?
Is A-VD_{O_2} over 1.0 vol, % above
baseline value (at zero PEEP)?

ALL NO

ANY YES

Terminate study:
Repeat observations at zero PEEP
Select PEEP setting with best Pa_{O_2}
Reduce FI_{O_2} in steps until Pa_{O_2}
is 60-65 mm Hg

Watch for pneumothorax
Limits of algorithm
Consult other sources
END

Has Pa_{O_2} fallen >5 mm below baseline
Pa_{O_2}?
Has Pa_{CO_2} risen 5 mm above baseline
Pa_{CO_2}?

ALL NO

ANY YES

Is PEEP now 15 cm H_2O ?

YES

NO

The application of PEEP

Introduction PEEP is used to increase the oxygenation of the arterial blood. It accomplishes this by maintaining in the alveoli and airways a pressure greater than atmospheric pressure at the resting expiratory level. This end-expiratory pressure increases the functional residual capacity by reinflating collapsed alveoli. Positive end-expiratory pressure is created by maintaining a resistance to exhalation and may be applied with or without a ventilator.

Methods of application Many of the newer ventilators have built-in PEEP, which is applied by keeping the exhalation valve inflated throughout the expiratory phase with a pressure equal to the amount of PEEP desired.

Several devices that use an adjustable, spring-loaded diaphragm attached to the exhalation tubing are available. These devices may be used with or without a ventilator and are especially useful for delivering high levels of PEEP (greater than 30 cm H_2O).

Other available devices consist of a plastic cylinder containing a ball-valve or dead-weight mechanism of sufficient weight to occlude the orifice when the pressure in the expiratory tubing drops to a given level. These devices are commonly available in sizes of 2.5, 5, 10, and 15 cm H_2O and may be used in combinations to achieve the desired PEEP. They may be used with or without a ventilator.

The classic method of applying PEEP is to extend the exhalation tubing into a container of water 1 cm for every cm H_2O of PEEP desired.

A more recent form of this method is to rest a column of water on a rubber diaphragm that occludes two ports—one entry and one exit. The exhalation tubing is attached to the entry port, and the exhaled gas must then lift the column of water to reach the exit port. The level of the column of water equals the amount of PEEP applied.

Applying PEEP with resuscitation bags is discussed on p. 105.

Cautions In some ventilators with built-in PEEP, the amount of PEEP applied will change as other settings are changed.

Ball-valve or dead-weight devices must be kept in the upright position to maintain PEEP.

When expiratory flow rates are high, water-column devices are subject to the problems of evaporation and spillage, which cause a decrease in PEEP.

Spring-loaded diaphragm devices must be checked periodically for wear and calibration.

Most PEEP devices have a retard effect on exhalation that increases as the amount of PEEP is increased. At rapid respiratory rates this may become evident as a slightly higher PEEP level than was established, because exhalation is not completed before the next inspiration begins.

Pneumothorax PEEP increases MIP. A high MIP appears to increase the risk pf pneumothorax. Equipment for treating pneumothorax should be assembled and available before a PEEP study is begun.

Comments on the PEEP algorithm

```
┌─────────────────────────────┐        ┌─────────────────────────────┐
│ Can Pa_O2 > 60 be achieved  │        │ Is patient known to be      │
│      with F_IO2 < 0.5?      │        │ adapted to Pa_O2 this       │
│                             │        │ low (e.g., COPD)?           │
└─────────────────────────────┘        └─────────────────────────────┘
```

One goal of ventilator therapy is to maintain a Pa_{O_2} of 60 mm Hg or more using an $F_{I_{O_2}}$ of 0.5 or less. If a concentration of oxygen higher than 0.5 is required, PEEP should be considered, since oxygen toxicity will result in approximately 24 to 48 hours with the use of $F_{I_{O_2}}$s over 0.5.

If a patient is chronically hypoxemic ($Pa_{O_2} \sim 50$ mm Hg) adaptation to this condition has probably occurred, and neither PEEP nor high concentrations of oxygen should be used to increase the Pa_{O_2} unless other indications exist.

```
┌──────────────────────────┐
│   Is V_T < 15 ml/kg?     │
└──────────────────────────┘
```

Diseased and collapsed alveoli can sometimes be reexpanded or kept open by using large tidal volumes and intermittent sigh volumes. Before the use of PEEP is considered, the tidal volume should be increased in steps to 15 ml/kg while the blood gas levels are being monitored.

```
┌──────────────────────────┐
│   Does systolic BP fall  │
│   >15 mm Hg during       │
│   inspiration?           │
└──────────────────────────┘
```

Fluctuations in blood pressure, particularly systolic levels, may well indicate hypovolemia or cardiac dysfunction. If either or both of these situations exist, they will be aggravated by the addition of PEEP. These problems should be corrected prior to the initiation of PEEP.

```
┌──────────────────────────┐
│   Is PAW >18 mm Hg?      │
└──────────────────────────┘
```

Left ventricular failure may be aggravated by the use of PEEP. Careful evaluation of the circulatory system and the heart should be carried out prior to the use of PEEP.

```
┌──────────────────────────┐
│  Prepare for PEEP study  │
│                          │
│   Set F_IO2 at 1.0       │
│                          │
│   Have chest tubes,      │
│   Pleurovac, and         │
│   instruments at         │
│   bedside                │
│                          │
│   Start PEEP study       │
│   flow sheet             │
└──────────────────────────┘
```

The determination of the "best PEEP" is most accurately done in steps and with the patient breathing 100% oxygen for 20 minutes. Having the chest tube insertion equipment at hand minimizes the amount of time required for the insertion of a chest tube should a pneumothorax develop. Finally, carefully recording on a form the values obtained during the study will assure access to the data required to make the determination of "best PEEP."

```
Obtain baseline
values for BP, MIP,
ABG, A-VD_{O_2}, and
static pressure
```

PEEP may have an adverse effect on blood pressure, MIP, Pa_{O_2}, or cardiac output. Since the ventilator patient is sick already, it is necessary to establish baseline values for comparison.

```
Add 5 cm H_2O PEEP
```

The application of PEEP is discussed elsewhere. It is important to measure the level of PEEP in a consistent manner and to do so on a regular basis, since various factors can change the delivered PEEP. It is always best to start with 5 cm H_2O and work upwards.

```
Observe 3-5 minutes
```

```
Measure MIP, static pressure, V_T,
BP, HR, observe rhythm
```

```
Does MIP exceed 50 cm H_2O?
Does MIP now exceed MIP at previous
  setting by more than 10 cm H_2O?
```

```
Did static pressure rise by more than
5 cm H_2O with current PEEP setting?
```

At each step, the maximum inspiratory pressure should not increase more than the amount of PEEP added—5 cm H_2O. If it does, one needs to differentiate between increased airway resistance caused by bronchoconstriction and decreased lung compliance. Follow the algorithm to determine what the best course of action is, according to the changes in maximum inspiratory and/or static pressure.

```
Does systolic BP drop >15 mm Hg.
during inspiration?
```

The increase in intrathoracic pressure and/or compression of the heart may lead to decreased cardiac output. If this happens, it may be reflected in a blood pressure drop. If PEEP causes blood pressure to fall, the cardiac and circulatory systems should be evaluated and their functions improved before proceeding with PEEP.

```
After 20 minutes obtain and submit
arterial and mixed venous blood for
Pa_{O_2}, Pa_{CO_2},
and O_2 content
```

```
Is A-VD_{O_2} more than 6.0 vol % ?
Is A-VD_{O_2} over 1.0 vol % above
baseline value (at zero PEEP)?
```

If this happens, the implication is that cardiac function has been impaired by the current level of PEEP. The study should be terminated, and the best PEEP should be selected by examining the results of the previous steps in the study.

```
Has Pa_{O_2} fallen >5 mm below baseline
Pa_{O_2}?
Has Pa_{CO_2} risen >5 mm above baseline
Pa_{CO_2}?
```

If either of the above has occurred, PEEP is working to the patient's disadvantage. The study should be terminated and the best PEEP selected by using the results of the previous steps in the study.

```
Is PEEP now 15 cm H_2O ?
```

All the steps are repeated until three levels of PEEP—5, 10 and 15 cm H_2O—have been tested with all measurements taken or until the limits of the algorithm have been exceeded. Observations are made again on zero PEEP. The best PEEP is the one that produces the best level of Pa_{O_2}.

Adjusting PEEP

Introduction This section addresses the decisions that need to be made when adjustment of PEEP is being considered. It is assumed that PEEP has been initiated according to the guidelines provided in the PEEP algorithm. It is also assumed that PEEP is being used so that the F_{IO_2} can be reduced while an acceptable level of Pa_{O_2} is maintained.

Principles As the patient improves, F_{IO_2} is reduced.

PEEP may be reduced below original level when:
    The F_{IO_2} is 0.5 or less (unless PEEP algorithm limits are exceeded previously)
    The Pa_{O_2} is 90 mm Hg on current setting of F_{IO_2}
    The patient has been stable in all other respects (BP, HR, rhythm, and PEEP setting) for 12 hours

PEEP should be reduced in steps of 5 cm H_2O or less.

Goal The goal is to decrease the PEEP level while maintaining a Pa_{O_2} of at least 60 mm Hg on an F_{IO_2} of 0.5 or less.

Procedure
1. Evaluate the situation:
   a. Is the F_{IO_2} 0.5 or less?
   b. Has the patient been stable for 12 hours or more?
   c. Is the current Pa_{O_2} 90 mm Hg or more?
2. If all answers to these questions are yes, decrease PEEP by 5 cm H_2O.
3. Continuously observe the patient for:
   a. BP, HR, rhythm
   b. Respiratory rate and amount of work required for breathing
4. If any observations are unacceptable:
   a. Draw ABG sample immediately
   b. Resume previous PEEP setting
   c. Evaluate ABG sample. If Pa_{O_2} is 90 or more, investigate for other causes of adverse effects. Wait until the patient has stabilized, and reevaluate
5. If no adverse effects are noted, obtain and evaluate ABG sample after 20 minutes.
6. If the Pa_{O_2} is 60 or greater on the new PEEP setting:
   a. Maintain new PEEP level for 12 hours
   b. Then reevaluate for further reduction of PEEP

A-V$_{DO_2}$ If a pulmonary artery line is in place, obtain a baseline A-V$_{DO_2}$ and repeat with each PEEP change.

When to retreat Adjusting PEEP can cause physiologic changes in cardiac function. If the A-V$_{DO_2}$ has dropped to unacceptable levels (to more than 6 vol% or by more than 1 vol%), PEEP should be resumed at original levels until cardiac function is stable. If an A-V$_{D_{O_2}}$ is not available, other indicators of cardiac function should be watched carefully.

If the Pa$_{O_2}$ drops below 60 mm Hg, the most prudent course is to resume original levels of PEEP.

If the patient is exhibiting signs of exhaustion (for example, increase in respiratory rate, increased use of accessory muscles, arrhythmias, tachycardia, or increased blood pressure), resume original levels of PEEP.

Some patients may exhibit signs of fatigue even though the Pa$_{O_2}$ is acceptable. Look for other causes of fatigue.

Success   If the Pa$_{O_2}$ does not drop below 60 and no other signs of distress appear, maintain the patient on the new level of PEEP, and repeat the evaluation.

Comments   The guidelines that have been presented are intentionally conservative. To the extent possible, the guidelines are based on objective clinical measurements or observations rather than "clinical judgment" or "experience."

Some patients are easier to "wean" from PEEP than others. For this group of patients, the team should feel free to accelerate the process that has been described.

CHAPTER 22

Weaning

Evaluation of readiness

Introduction   Most patients who have required a ventilator for fewer than 2 days can be weaned quickly and simply. Patients who have been sick and dependent on the ventilator longer will adjust more slowly. Some techniques for facilitating this adjustment are described.

Perspective   There are probably several acceptable ways to wean a patient. The guidelines that follow are designed for the MD, the RN, and the RT who are beginners at weaning. The guidelines are intentionally conservative. To the extent possible, they are based on specific objective clinical measurements or observations rather than "clinical judgment" or "experience."

Types of patients

Short termers

Some patients seem ready for weaning after only 1 or 2 days of ventilation. Since such patients are usually easy to wean, the procedure described below may be too slow. For this group of patients, the team should feel free to accelerate the weaning process.

Long termers

Patients attached to a ventilator more than 3 days are harder to wean because the muscles of respiration become deconditioned. Also, the diseases that make ventilation of these patients necessary are usually more serious and require more time to resolve. The guidelines that follow are aimed at this group.

Think weaning each afternoon   As soon as you have solved the problems involved in beginning to ventilate a patient, start thinking about how you are going to stop ventilating him. We recommend that late every afternoon (for example, at 1700 hours [5:00]), the team regularly and deliberately review the patient's readiness for weaning.

Why each afternoon?   Such a daily routine means that the decision to wean will be made as early as possible. Making the decision late in the afternoon permits the team to schedule the weaning process to follow a good night's rest. Patients are easier to wean if they are rested.

How does the team decide to wean? First, the team should determine if the patient has any drive to breathe. Next, the team should consider whether the heart and thorax are ready for the stress of weaning. The team should also review any current difficulties with oxygenation and ventilation.

Is the patient triggering? Usually the first step in weaning is to allow the patient to trigger the ventilator. This permits the patient to demonstrate his drive to breathe and to set his own blood gas goals.

Is the heart ready? Weaning places stress on at least two structures—the heart and the chest wall. If the cardiovascular system is not compensated or stabilized, weaning can only make matters worse. Usually weaning should be deferred until cardiovascular problems have been minimized. This is obviously a clinical judgment. How to make this judgment is beyond the scope of these guidelines.

Is the chest wall stable? The stability of the chest wall should be evaluated. If a flail segment or a recent thoractomy has not yet stabilized, weaning will only make matters worse. This is another clinical judgment.

Is weaning too much work? The readiness of the respiratory muscles to provide the effort required can be evaluated by some measurements of lung mechanics. The following criteria should be satisfied before attempting weaning:

f less than 25 BPM (during mechanical ventilation)
Peak pressure (during mechanical ventilation) less than 30 cm H_2O
Inspiratory force greater than -20 cm H_2O
VC greater than 15 ml/kg (unless known to be previously impaired; for example, if patient has COPD, use VC greater than 10 ml/kg)

What is the Pa_{O_2}? Weaning should be deferred until Pa_{O_2} is greater than 60 on an FI_{O_2} less than 0.5.

Minimize other problems To the extent possible, other problems should be minimized the evening before weaning. Consider the following:

Depressed consciousness
Depressed cough
Excess pulmonary secretions
Atelectasis
Bronchospasm
Fever
Electrolyte imbalances
Abdominal distention
Anemia

Metabolic acidosis

Anxiety

Reevaluate at 0730 hours (7:30 AM) In the morning, before weaning the patient, review once more his readiness to wean:

Has his cardiovascular status deteriorated during the night?

Has he become more difficult to ventilate or oxygenate?

Have other problems developed?

Weaning procedure

Introduction This procedure assumes that the patient's readiness for weaning has been evaluated in accordance with the guidelines previously described.

Prepare the patient Before weaning the patient, explain to him exactly what you will be doing. Reassure the patient that you will not leave his side. Explain that you must find out how much he can do on his own, and enlist his cooperation in a 20-minute test. Allow the patient to assume a comfortable position. Sit him up if possible. If you feel that the patient might splint his chest because of pain, consider administering small doses of morphine sulfate prior to weaning.

Challenge the patient Try having the patient use a T piece (blow-by). Maintain the same $F_{I_{O_2}}$, and monitor at 5-minute intervals.

Monitor the patient's response Measure and record the patient's heart rate, blood pressure, and respiratory rate at least every 5 minutes. Make sure the patient can let you know if he experiences:

Dyspnea

Fatigue

Panic

Pain

Observe the patient for:

Labored breathing

Sweating

Arrhythmias

Restlessness

Drowsiness

Flaring of ala nasi

Intercostal retractions

Use of accessory muscles of respiration

Abort procedure *If* the patient experiences more distress than he is willing to tolerate, *or*

The respiratory rate exceeds 25, or drops to below 8, *or*

Systolic blood pressure drops 20 mm Hg or rises 30 mm Hg, *or*

Pulse rate rises by more than 20 beats per minute, *or*

Premature ventricular contractions (PVC) exceed 4 per minute, *or*

Patient makes increasing use of accessory muscles of respiration,

131

Then assure the patient that you will discontinue the test within 1 minute.
> Draw arterial blood sample to determine gas levels
> Restore ventilator settings as before challenge
> Evaluate blood gas test results
> Consider rechallenge in 1 to 2 hours

Successful trial *If* the abort procedure is not activated within 20 minutes, *then* measure vital capacity
> Draw arterial blood samples to determine gas levels
> Restore ventilator settings as before challenge
> Allow patient to rest 1 hour

Keep trying T piece Keep challenging the patient to use the T piece for longer and longer periods. Allow each trial to continue until the patient exceeds abort criteria. Allow the patient to rest one hour while being ventilated, and try the T piece again. Keep trying until the patient can tolerate the T piece for 4 hours. Then consider extubation. If the patient is not ready for extubation by 2000 hours (8:00 PM), discontinue trials and return the patient to assisted ventilation for the night.

Consider extubation *If* the patient has used the T piece for 4 hours and
> f is less than 25
> VC is greater than 15 ml/kg
> Pa_{O_2} is greater than 60 on FI_{O_2} less than 0.5
> Pa_{CO_2} is less than 45 (or pH is greater than 7.35)
> Vital signs remain stable

Then consider proceeding according to the section on extubation.

Setbacks or tough cases If the abort procedure is repeatedly activated at early stages of the weaning process, be prepared to improvise an even more gradual weaning schedule.

The transition from controlled ventilation to T piece can be made more gradual by switching the patient to a pressure-cycled ventilator or using intermittent demand ventilation (IDV). A patient can often tolerate 30 to 60 minutes of spontaneous ventilation before showing signs of fatigue. However, if the patient is allowed to continue another hour or two, he will exhaust himself and may need continuous ventilation for a full day to recover. In such patients, it is better to try regular short periods of spontaneous ventilation with periodic ventilator assistance than to "go for broke."

Extubation

We will now consider extubation following weaning. It should be established that the patient is not likely to require mechanical ventilation in the next 24 hours.

Need for airway At this point, the team should consider the possibility that the patient may still need an airway for other reasons. These include:

> Access to secretions (for example, poor cough, excess secretions)
> Prevention of aspiration (for example, obtunded condition, poor gag reflex)
> Narrow airway (for example, trauma to face or neck)

In such cases extubation might be delayed or coordinated with tracheostomy.

Procedure The following procedure for extubation is suggested. Observe cardiac rhythm throughout the procedure.

1. Place the patient in a high Fowler's position.
2. Preoxygenate and hyperinflate with a resuscitator bag.
3. Suction through an endotracheal tube.
4. Oxygenate and hyperventilate.
5. Suction the pharynx.
6. Loosen the tape supporting the endotracheal tube.
7. Oxygenate and hyperinflate.
8. Advance the suction catheter down the endotracheal tube.
   Release air from the cuff quickly.
   Suction while withdrawing the endotracheal tube.

   > *or*

   Deflate the cuff.
   Pull the tube, asking the patient to cough while it is being removed.
9. Have the patient cough and take deep breaths.
10. Administer the same $F_{I_{O_2}}$ as prior to extubation.
11. Observe the patient carefully, encouraging him to take deep breaths and cough.
12. Measure BP, pulse, and f every 10 min for 3 times.
13. Observe the patient continuously for 30 minutes for signs of respiratory distress.
14. Measure ABG levels after 30 minutes.
15. Adjust $F_{I_{O_2}}$ according to ABG levels.
16. Initiate routine patient monitoring and care as appropriate.

PART THREE

Exercises

Learning goals for the exercises

Introduction   Some students (and instructors) are more comfortable if they can work toward learning goals. Some key learning goals of Part III are listed below. The goals are listed in the order in which they have been discussed in this book.

Indications for intubation and ventilation

1. Given a series of descriptions of clinical situations, the student will select those situations in which the patient is at high risk of progressive respiratory failure and cite a reason. The guidelines included in this book will be used to evaluate the student's response.

2. Given the f, VC, Pa_{O_2}, Pa_{CO_2}, and pH in any of the above high-risk situations, the student will determine whether mechanical ventilation is indicated. The guidelines included in the book will be used to evaluate the student's responses.

Airway selection

3. Given a series of clinical situations involving patients attached to ventilators, the student will select the most suitable airway. The guidelines in the book will be used to determine the preferred airway.

4. Given an endotracheal tube with the low-pressure cuff in place in a patient (or model) attached to a ventilator, the student will inflate the cuff with a volume of air just sufficient to control leakage.

5. Given a series of tubes with cuffs of different degrees of compliance, the student will select the cuffs with higher degrees of compliance.

Selection of ventilator

6. Given a list of the ventilators in use in the student's hospital, the student will name the ventilators and classify them as pressure-cycled or volume-cycled.

7. Given descriptions of common situations in which mechanical ventilation is indicated, the student will determine whether a pressure-cycled or a volume-cycled ventilator is preferred. The algorithm provided in the book will be used to determine the preferred ventilator.

Ventilator readiness

8. Given a complete ventilator system, a spirometer, a test lung, and an appropriate checklist, the student will determine whether:
    a. Humidifier is functioning
    b. Inspired gas temperature is 37 C
    c. System is free of leaks
    d. Spirometer is functioning
    e. Alarms are functioning
    The student will complete this task in 5 minutes.

Initial settings

9. Given an operational ventilator, a spirometer, an oxygen analyzer, a test lung, and the weight of a hypothetical patient, the student will adjust the ventilator so that the f, V_T, I:E ratio, $F_{I_{O_2}}$, and sensitivity correspond to guidelines provided in this book.

Management 10. Given a simulated patient attached to a ventilator, an interdisciplinary (MD, RN, and RT) team of students will be able to:
a. Adjust the $\dot{V}E$ and FI_{O_2} in response to blood gas data
b. Bag, suction, and/or deep breathe the patient in accordance with checklists included in the book
c. Carry out routine monitoring procedures and preventive measures described in the book

Weaning 11. Given clinical summaries complete with results of blood gas analysis and spirometry, the student will indicate which patients may be ready for weaning trials.

12. Given a patient attached to a ventilator and other appropriate equipment, the student will set up a T piece (blow-by), disconnect the patient from the ventilator, and connect the T piece to the patient.

13. Given a patient doing well with a T piece, the student will extubate the patient in accordance with the procedure included in this book.

PEEP 14. Given data from PEEP studies in progress (but not yet completed), the student will indicate whether the study should be continued and the next PEEP setting or measurement employed.

15. Given a ventilator, PEEP setup, and test lung, the student will make the adjustments necessary to achieve any PEEP value between 0 and 20 cm H_2O while maintaining $\dot{V}$ constant and MIP less than 50 cm H_2O.

EXERCISE 1

Ventilometrics exercise

This exercise is designed to give the student an opportunity to apply key ventilometric concepts.

The student is provided with a pressure/volume time tracing. The student is asked to make measurements and derive values.

An annotated instructor version is also provided.

Student version

How much information can you obtain about the patient-ventilator system from this graph?

(Assume the patient is attached to an MA-1 ventilator)

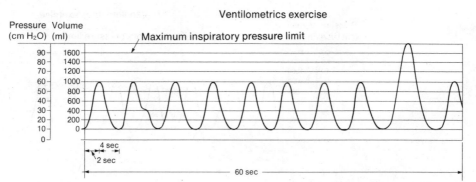

Ventilometrics exercise

Respiratory rate _____

Tidal volume _____

Inspiratory pressure _____

Sigh volume _____

Sigh frequency _____

Sigh multiple _____

Is all of the sigh delivered? _____

I : E ratio _____

Mean inspiratory flow _____

Static pressure _____

Dynamic compliance _____

Static compliance _____

End-expiratory pressure _____

Does the sigh alter the respiratory rate? ____

Does inflation hold affect mean airway pressure? _____

Probable cause of high inspiratory pressure?

    Lung compliance? _____

    Airway resistance? _____

Do any of these adjustments affect the I : E ratio?

    Tidal volume _____

    Respiratory rate _____

    Inspiratory flow _____

    PEEP _____

Instructor version

How much information can you obtain about the patient-ventilator system from this graph?

(Assume the patient is attached to an MA-1 ventilator)

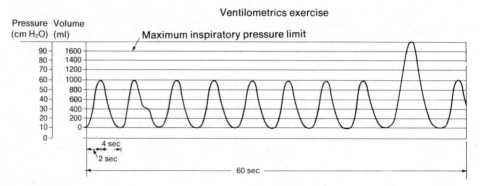

Ventilometrics exercise

Respiratory rate ___10___

Tidal volume ___1000 ml___

Inspiratory pressure ___60 cm H₂O___

Sigh volume ___1500 ml___

Sigh frequency ___1/min___

Sigh multiple ___1___

Is all of the sigh delivered? ___No___

I:E ratio ___1:2___

Mean inspiratory flow ___30 LPM___

Static pressure ___30 cm H₂O___

Dynamic compliance ___20 ml/cm H₂O___

Static compliance ___50 ml/cm H₂O___

End-expiratory pressure ___+10 cm H₂O___

Does the sigh alter the respiratory rate? ___Yes___

Does inflation hold affect mean airway pressure? ___Yes___

Probable cause of high inspiratory pressure?

Lung compliance? ___No___

Airway resistance ? ___Yes___

Do any of these adjustments affect the I:E ratio?

Tidal volume ___Yes___

Respiratory rate ___Yes___

Inspiratory flow ___Yes___

PEEP ___No___

Endotracheal tube exercise

Overview This exercise is for each member of the team involved in the care of patients who are candidates for continuous ventilation.

Target group The target group is comprised of MDs, RNs, and RTs who are responsible for the insertion of airways or the care of patients with artificial airways in place.

Setting An appropriate setting is a conference room or other large workroom with tables for spreading out equipment and chairs for the students.

Pretest Before beginning this exercise, the student should be able to demonstrate proper intubation technique, state indications for and hazards of endotracheal intubation, and describe the desirable characteristics of endotracheal and tracheostomy tubes.

Objectives At the conclusion of the session the student will be able to:
1. Select, from an assortment of tubes, one that most nearly meets optimal criteria
2. Select an airway of the appropriate size to fit a model trachea
3. Intubate successfully an intubation mannikin
4. Inflate the cuff of the tube to "just seal," using a cuff inflation gauge while ventilating the mannikin at a variety of inflation pressures
5. Select a suction catheter of the appropriate size for the airway used
6. Demonstrate proper suctioning technique, including hyperinflation and hyperoxygenation before and after suctioning

Time frame This exercise will last 60 to 90 minutes, depending on the number of students and their degrees of expertise.

Materials
1. Intubation mannikin that can be ventilated with a bag or ventilator
2. Assortment of endotracheal and tracheostomy tubes of different types and sizes
3. Assortment of suction kits of different types and sizes
4. Resuscitation bag and oxygen source
5. Pressure ventilator

6. Cuff inflation pressure gauge
7. Model tracheas of different sizes, preferably clear and flexible
8. Suction source
9. Laryngoscope with assortment of curved and straight blades
10. Suctioning procedure instructions
11. Selection-of-airway procedure instructions

Lesson plan
1. Prearrange the equipment in the following order:
   a. Cuff pressure gauge, assortment of airways and artificial tracheas
   b. Laryngoscope and selection of blades
   c. Suction source and assortment of suction kits
   d. Intubation mannikin
   e. Ventilator, resuscitation bag, and oxygen source (ventilator resuscitator bag should be assembled and ready for use)
2. The students should begin by testing and selecting an airway, proceeding to each station, and selecting the appropriate device, and finish by successfully intubating, ventilating, suctioning, and hyperinflating the mannikin.*
3. The instructor should remain in the room to act as a resource person.
4. After practice, this exercise should be repeated, using first an anesthetized animal in an animal laboratory and then, if possible, a surgical patient in the operating room.

*If time permits, the intracuff pressure should be measured at the "minimal leak" and "just seal" inflations for each of the high-volume low-pressure and low-volume high-pressure cuffs.

EXERCISE 3

Self-guided tours of ventilators

Overview This is a "hands-on" introductory session on ventilators. In each tour, the student uses a set of self-guiding instructions to become familiar with the operational aspects of one ventilator. Parallel versions are presented for the following models: Bird, Ohio 560, Searle VVA, and Bennett MA-1.

Target group The target group is comprised of MDs, RNs, and RTs involved in the care of patients requiring continuous mechanical ventilation.

Objectives At the conclusion of this session, the student will be able to:
1. Indicate and operate all adjustable parameters necessary to properly ventilate a patient with the specified ventilator.
2. Indicate and demonstrate all safety devices of the specified ventilator.
3. Explain and demonstrate appropriate manual methods of monitoring the effectiveness of ventilation.

Time frame This exercise will last 60 to 90 minutes.

Setting A good setting is a private room with a 110-volt electrical outlet and 50 PSI sources of oxygen and air.

Materials
1. Specified ventilator with manifold and tubing
2. In-circuit monitoring spirometer
3. Test lung
4. Manual spirometer (Wright or Draeger)
5. Oxygen analyzer
6. Chronometer
7. Self-guiding instructions

Pretest No pretest is required.

Lesson plan
1. Explain to the students how the self-guided tour works. Any exceptionally knowledgeable member of the student team may act as a resource person.
2. Explain abbreviations and terms that might be used.
3. Allow the students to proceed through the worksheets without prompting, but remain nearby to answer questions. Students may work in pairs.

Post-test No post-test is required. The instructor will have sufficient opportunity during the exercise to observe the speed with which the student completes a module and the number of difficulties encountered requiring assistance. The exercise's emphasis on the recurrent use of most of the parameters, alarms, and monitoring methods also allows for ongoing evaluation.

Self-guided tour of the Bird ventilator

This is one of four similar modules, each of which concentrates on a different ventilator.

This hands-on exercise is designed to familiarize the student with the ventilator controls, displays, and mechanics.

Students usually work in pairs. Each pair proceeds at its own pace. An instructor is on call nearby.

One instructor can supervise three pairs.

Objectives The student will establish V_T, I : E ratio, sensitivity, flow rate, and f on the Bird ventilator.

The student will verify settings by using a spirometer and an oxygen analyzer.

The student will record measurements on a ventilator flow sheet.

Equipment required
1. Bird Mark VII, VIII, X, or XIV ventilator
2. Rubber test lung*
3. Wright and Draeger spirometer
4. Ventilator flow sheet
5. Bird circuit
6. Chronometer

Skills required
1. Ability to use spirometer
2. Ability to use oxygen analyzer
3. Ability to measure I : E ratio

TO INSTRUCTORS: All controls should be in "off" or minimal-setting positions.

Tasks

☐ 1. Review locations of all controls
   ☐ Inspiratory sensitivity effort
   ☐ Pressure gauge
   ☐ Inspiratory time flow rate
   ☐ Air-mix
   ☐ Expiratory time for apnea
   ☐ Inspiratory pressure limit
☐ 2. Turn inspiratory flow rate control to zero
☐ 3. Lock air-mix control in "out" position
☐ 4. Connect high pressure oxygen hose to 50 PSI oxygen source
☐ 5. Connect patient circuit to ventilator and test lung to patient circuit

*The test lung should have a reasonably stiff compliance and have the compliance band intact.

Setting respiratory rate

☐ 6. Set the ventilator as follows:

$$\text{Sensitivity} = 10$$
$$\text{Flow rate} = 25$$
$$\text{Pressure} = 15$$
$$f = 10$$

Adjust apnea control (turn counterclockwise) to achieve f of 10
Measure f with chronometer

f = _____

Comments:

If numbers exist on the apnea control, they are reference points
  only. They are not breaths per minute or time in seconds.

Apnea control is used *only* for patients who do not have an adequate
  respiratory rate.

The apnea control should be in the "off" position for treatments.

Simulating assisted ventilation

☐ 7. Turn apnea control to "off" position
  Set sensitivity at 5
  Squeeze and abruptly release test lung
  Watch inspiratory pressure gauge during this maneuver

Comments:

With each squeeze, the needle moves into the negative (pink) pressure zone, simulating a patient-initiated breath.

The lower the number, the easier for the patient to start the next
  breath.

Calibration of this control may not be precise. Watch the patient's
  effort in breathing and the pressure gauge rather than relying on
  the number.

Most patients breathe comfortably with a -1 to -2 cm H_2O effort.

If the setting is too sensitive, it can self-cycle the ventilator.

Simulating controlled ventilation

☐ 8. Keep apnea control in "off" position
  Set sensitivity at 50
  Squeeze and abruptly release test lung
  Watch inspiratory pressure gauge during this maneuver

Comments:

You should not be able to trigger a breath with this maneuver. This
  sensitivity setting is for controlled ventilation.

If a breath can be triggered, the sensitivity control needs calibration.

☐ 9. Set sensitivity at 5

Adjust apnea control to achieve f of 6

Between automatically triggered breaths, squeeze and abruptly release test lung

Comment: To guarantee a minimum number of breaths, set a slow
base rate for patients who may become apneic.

Setting the I:E ratio

☐ 10. Set the ventilator as follows:

Sensitivity = 10
Pressure = 15
Flow rate = 40
f = 16

Determine I:E ratio

At IFR 40 I:E ratio = _____

Change flow rate to 25

At IFR 25 I:E ratio = _____

Change flow rate to 10

At IFR 10 I:E ratio = _____

Comments:

The flow rate is the speed at which gas *flows* into the test lung (or
patient).

The flow rate determines the length of time required for inspiration.

The I:E ratio may change whenever flow, pressure, apnea control,
or the patient's lung compliance changes. Whenever you are adjusting any controls, check the I:E ratio that results.

Setting and determining the maximum inspiratory pressure

☐ 11. Set the ventilator as follows:

Sensitivity = 15
Flow rate = 10
Pressure = 15
f = 10

Measure V_T

V_T = _____

Note MIP on pressure gauge

MIP = _____

Note I:E ratio

I:E ratio = _____

Change pressure to 10
Measure V_T

V_T = _____

Note MIP on pressure gauge

MIP = _____

Change pressure to 25
Measure V_T

V_T = _____

Note MIP on pressure gauge

MIP = _____

Questions:
Does V_T increase or decrease with an increase in pressure?
Does f change with a change in pressure? If so, why?
Does the I:E ratio change with a change in pressure? If so, why?

Comment: The I:E ratio may change whenever flow, pressure, apnea control interval, or the patient's lung compliance changes. Whenever you are adjusting any controls, check the I:E ratio that results.

Altering settings

☐ 12. Set sensitivity at 10

Adjust appropriate settings to achieve:

V_T = 800 ml
I:E ratio = 1:2
f = 12

Verify each value

Question: What controls did you use?

☐ 13. Push air-mix knob in
Measure V_T

V_T measured = _____

Measure I:E ratio

I:E ratio = _____

Measure f

f = _____

Question: Did any of the values change? Why?

Comments:

With this knob pushed in, the gas supply to the ventilator comes from your high pressure gas source only. No room air is entrained along with the oxygen for delivery to the lung. Flow is limited to oxygen only.

Because the flow is decreased, the inspiratory time lengthens, and the respiratory rate drops.

☐ 14. Turn flow rate to "off"

Disconnect high pressure oxygen hose and secure to ventilator

Self-guided tour of the Ohio 560 ventilator

This is one of four similar modules, each of which concentrates on a different ventilator.

This hands-on exercise is designed to familiarize the student with the ventilator controls, displays, and mechanics.

Students usually work in pairs. Each pair proceeds at its own pace. An instructor is on call nearby.

One instructor can supervise three pairs.

Objectives The student will establish V_T, f, I:E ratio, sigh volume, frequency of sigh, FI_{O_2}, and level of patient triggering effort.

The student will enable and disable alarms at a variety of settings.

The student will verify settings by using a spirometer and an oxygen analyzer.

The student will record measurements on a ventilator flow sheet.

Equipment required
1. Ohio 560 ventilator
2. Rubber test lung*
3. Wright or Draeger spirometer
4. Oxygen analyzer
5. Ventilator flow sheet
6. Patient circuit
7. Chronometer

Skills required
1. Ability to use spirometer
2. Ability to use oxygen analyzer
3. Ability to measure I:E ratio

TO INSTRUCTORS: The ventilator should have all controls in "off" or "disabled" positions and volumes at zero, *except* that pressure or volume alarms or "pop-offs" should be operative at maximum levels of pressure or volume.

The ventilator should *not* be plugged in or connected to oxygen.

Tasks

☐ 1. Review locations of the following:

Controls and signals
FI_{O_2} control
Deep breath interval
Manual deep breath
Humidifier output

---

*The test lung should have a reasonably stiff compliance and have the compliance band intact.

151

Inflation hold
Plateau (CPPB)
Patient triggering (light)
Patient triggering effort
Deep breath volume
Tidal volume
Patient resistance
Respiration rate (meter)
Expiration time (seconds)
Inspiratory flow
Manual inspiration/expiration
Power on/off
Alarms and safety features
All models
Oxygen alarm
Failure-to-cycle
Low pressure alarm light
Intermittent/continuous toggle switch
Reset alarm button
Pressure relief valve (under front panel)
Newer models
High pressure limit control
High pressure alarm light

☐ 2. Turn power switch off
☐ 3. Plug power cord into grounded 110-volt AC outlet
☐ 4. Connect high pressure oxygen hose directly to 50 PSI oxygen source
      (Do not connect to an oxygen flow meter)
☐ 5. Connect test lung to Y piece of patient circuit
☐ 6. Turn power switch on

Setting tidal volume

☐ 7. Adjust ventilator settings as follows:

$$V_T = 600 \text{ ml}$$
Expiratory time = 4
Inspiratory flow = 2

Measure expired V_T with spirometer

$V_T = $ *604 cc*

Question: Does this measurement agree with your setting? If not, why not?

Comments:
V_T should be set while watching the inflation bellows on a direct line (rather than at an angle), or you may be about 100 ml off (parallax error).

Inspiratory bellows are accurate only to ±50 ml.

Leaks may exist in the system.

Calibration of the spirometer may not be precise.

Placement of the spirometer may influence readings.

Setting respiratory rate

☐ 8. Leave V$_T$ at 600 ml

Adjust inspiratory flow and expiratory time settings as necessary to obtain respiratory rate of 20 to register on meter

Measure respiratory rate for 1 minute

f = _____ *20*

Questions:

Which controls did you use? *insp. flow ↓, ↓ exp. time*

Are they related?

Comment: Expiratory time is calibrated in seconds. The inspiratory flow setting is not calibrated. The numbers are reference points only.

Setting the I:E ratio

☐ 9. Leave V$_T$ at 600.

Maintain f at 20

Adjust expiratory time and inspiratory flow settings until you achieve I:E ratio of 1:2

Observing changes produced, manipulate controls that adjust I:E ratio until you are comfortable with their use

Comment: Timing with a stop watch or tapping out time increments is acceptable. "Breathing with" the ventilator to set the ratio generally leads to error.

Fine tuning

☐ 10. Adjust V$_T$ to 900 ml

Note effect on f and I:E ratio

Correct f to 20

Correct I:E ratio to 1:2

R.R.^{3} →J↑ ET↑

Questions:

What happens to the respiratory rate when expiratory time is increased or decreased? *ET↑ RR↓, ET↓ RR↑*

What happens to the I:E ratio when the inspiratory flow is increased or decreased?

If you are not comfortable manipulating these controls, practice by changing each one separately.

Monitoring maximum inspiratory pressure

☐ 11. Adjust settings as follows:

$$V_T = 600 \text{ ml}$$
$$f = 20$$
$$I:E \text{ ratio} = 1:2$$

Note patient resistance gauge

Record maximum inspiratory pressure

MIP = _32 cm H₂O_

Place alarm on intermittent

Lift front top panel from Ohio 560

Disconnect test lung

Occlude **Y** connector at end of tubing while adjusting internal pressure relief valve

In all models:

Set pressure relief valve so highest pressure reached during occlusion of tubing is about 15 cm H_2O greater than last observed MIP

Reconnect test lung

Enable alarm

Proceed to next step in exercise if your Ohio 560 model does not have an external high pressure alarm

In newer models, also set external high pressure alarm by depressing high pressure alarm and rotating until alarm pressure is about 10 cm H_2O higher than MIP

Kink inspiratory tubing sharply

Observe patient resistance gauge

MIP = _50 cm/H₂O_

Comments:

The MIP is equal to the sum of the resistance in the ventilator tubing and the test lung.

The pop-off control is usually set 10 to 15 cm H_2O higher than the MIP. However, if the MIP is over 50 cm H_2O, then the pop-off setting should be ordered by the physician.

The maximum inspiratory pressure will rise with sigh volumes.

If the pop-off control is set too low, the full sigh volume will not be delivered.

Setting sigh volumes

☐ 12. Set V_T bellows at 600 ml

Set sigh bellows at 600 ml

Attach reference spirometer to measure expired volumes

Use "manual deep breath" control to produce a sigh

Measure sigh volume

V_{sigh} = _____

Comments:

The sigh volume is the sum of the volume set in both bellows.

Hence, if the V_T bellows is set at 600 ml and the sigh bellows at 600 ml, the sigh volume should be 1200 ml.

If the sigh volume produces a maximum inspiratory pressure of 40 cm H_2O and the pop-off control is set at 30 cm H_2O, the preset sigh volume will not be delivered in full. Always set the pop-off control about 15 cm H_2O higher than the MIP normally produced with the sigh volume.

Maximum inspiratory pressures over 50 cm H_2O may be dangerous, and sigh volumes may need to be decreased if MIPs over 50 are generated.

Setting $F_{I_{O_2}}$

☐ 13. Insert oxygen analyzer between Y piece of the patient circuit and the test lung

Measure $F_{I_{O_2}}$ at each of the following settings:

$F_{I_{O_2}}$ setting	.21	.4	.6	1.0
Measured value				

Question: Do the measured values agree with the settings? If not, why not?

Comments:

Precise agreement requires accurate calibration of the oxygen analyzer. If the variance is within ±5%, the problem may be caused by either analyzer or ventilator error. Check the analyzer. (The ventilator is usually very stable within ±5%.)

If the variance is greater than ±5%, the analyzer must be recalibrated. Then recheck the $F_{I_{O_2}}$s. (Analyzer accuracy deteriorates with time.)

Patience is required. The response time of the ventilator to an $F_{I_{O_2}}$ change may be up to 60 seconds. This is an important point to remember if the ventilator setting is used to hyperoxygenate the patient prior to suctioning.

Altering settings

☐ 14. Set the ventilator as follows:

$$V_T = 900 \text{ ml}$$
$$F_{I_{O_2}} = .35$$
$$I:E \text{ ratio} = 1:2$$
$$f = 12$$

Sigh volume = 1500 ml
Deep breath interval = 8 min

Verify settings with spirometer, chronometer, and oyxgen analyzer
Observe patient resistance gauge (maximum pressure change)
Record all values on ventilator flow sheet

Set ventilator as follows:

V_T = 600 ml
f = 12
I:E ratio = 1:2

Verify settings with spirometer and chronometer
Observe patient resistance gauge
Record all values on ventilator flow sheet

Maintain f and I:E ratio
Set V_T to 400 ml
Verify settings with spirometer and chronometer
Observe patient resistance gauges
Record all values on ventilator flow sheet

Question: Do f and I:E ratio remain the same when V_T is changed? If not, why not?

Comment: Respiratory rate, I:E ratio, V_T, and inspiratory flow rate are interrelated. If the tidal volume is decreased but the inspiratory flow rate is kept the same, inflation will be completed in a shorter time. Each breath cycle will be shorter, more breaths will be completed in a minute, and thus, the respiratory rate will increase.

Simulating patient changes

☐ 15. Adjust ventilator controls as follows:

V_T = 700 ml
Sigh volume = 1200 ml
Deep breathing interval = 6 min
$F_{I_{O_2}}$ = 0.7
I:E ratio = 1:2
f = 10

Verify settings with monitoring equipment
Record all values on ventilator flow sheet
Change to smaller size of test lung (or manually occlude distal half of lung being used)
Observe any changes from what was just recorded on flow sheet

Comment: Decreasing the lung size (for example, by simulating mucus plugs or right main stem intubation) increases MIP.

Setting patient triggering effort

☐ 16. Set patient triggering-effort dial at "min" (if ventilator self-cycles, adjust setting until ventilator stops self-cycling)
Squeeze test lung and abruptly release while watching patient resistance gauge

Comments:
Note that a slight negative pressure is produced. The triggering light comes on, and the ventilator inflates the test lung.
With the setting in this position, it is easy for a patient to initiate breaths.

☐ 17. Set patient-triggering-effort dial at "max"
Squeeze test lung and abruptly release while watching patient resistance gauge

Comments:
It should be impossible to trigger a breath with this maneuver.
With the setting in this position, it is impossible for the patient to initiate breaths.

Functioning of alarms

☐ 18. Disconnect a tube in the inspiratory line
Note low pressure alarm signal
Disable alarm
Reconnect tube
Reset alarm

Use of inflation hold

☐ 19. Leave settings as in previous task
Observe movement of needle on airway pressure gauge; it should reach peak pressure, reverse rapidly, and return to zero
Turn inflation hold control to 2.0 seconds
Now note pause of needle at "end inspiration" (during this time, inhaled volume is held in lungs)
Turn inflation hold to zero

Comments:
For therapeutic purposes, this control is used *only* with a physician's orders.
This control may be used to measure static pressure.
There probably will be no change in static pressure noted if you are using a test lung.

Use of plateau

☐ 20. Turn plateau control to "max" while observing patient resistance gauge

Question: What is the effect produced?

Comments:
Never use plateau without a physician's order.
This control can set PEEP levels.

☐ 21. If you cannot answer questions or do not feel comfortable manipulating controls, seek help from instructor

☐ 22. Turn power switch off
Disconnect high pressure oxygen hose from oxygen source and secure to back of ventilator.
Disconnect power cord and secure to back of ventilator

Self-guided tour of the Searle VVA ventilator

This is one of four similar modules, each of which concentrates on a different ventilator.

This hands-on exercise is designed to familiarize the student with the ventilator controls, displays, and mechanics.

Students usually work in pairs. Each pair proceeds as its own pace. An instructor is on call nearby.

One instructor can supervise three pairs.

Objectives The student will establish V_T, f, I:E ratio, deep breath volume, frequency of deep breaths, $F_{I_{O_2}}$, and level of patient-triggering-effort and will enable and disable alarms at a variety of settings.

The student will verify settings by using a spirometer and an oxygen analyzer.

The student will record measurements on a ventilator flow sheet.

Equipment required
1. Searle VVA ventilator
2. Rubber test lung*
3. Wright or Draeger spirometer
4. Oxygen analyzer
5. Ventilator flow sheet
6. Patient circuit
7. Chronometer

Skills required
1. Ability to use spirometer
2. Ability to use oxygen analyzer
3. Ability to measure I:E ratio

TO INSTRUCTORS: The controls should be set as follows:
Spirometer warning level at zero
All ventilator controls on zero or minimal settings, except pressure alarm and
pressure relief set at 100 cm H_2O

Tasks

☐ 1. Review locations of the following controls and signals:

Ventilator
Inflation hold
O_2 concentration
Deep breath interval
Nebulizer
100% O_2
Multiple deep breath

*The test lung should have a reasonably stiff compliance and have the compliance band intact.

159

PEEP
Patient triggering effort
Patient triggering light
Deep breath volume
Tidal volume
Respiratory rate (digital)
Inspiratory flow taper
Inspiratory flow rate
I : E ratio (digital)
Airway pressure
Power
Manual deep breath
Manual inspiration
High inspiratory pressure warning
Inspiratory pressure relief
Press to test
Warning reset
Warning lights
Low inspiratory pressure
End-expiratory pressure
High inspiratory pressure
Inspiratory pressure relief
Short exhalation
Failure to cycle
Power disconnect
Low oxygen pressure
Fan
Spirometer (Autowedge spirometer)
Exhaled tidal volume (electronic, on top)
2-minute silence warning level
Exhaled tidal volume (mechanical, window)

☐ 2. Plug Searle VVA ventilator's power cord into grounded 110-volt AC outlet

☐ 3. Plug ventilator mode controller cord into grounded 110-volt AC outlet

☐ 4. Connect oxygen high pressure hose directly to 50 PSI oxygen source

☐ 5. Connect test lung to Y piece of patient circuit

☐ 6. Turn power switch on

Comments:

The fan alarm will stop after a few machine cycles. If it does not, check for dust in the filter.

Ignore all other alarms until settings in the next step are accomplished.

In all subsequent steps, if the V_T is changed while the ventilator is on, adjust the control *between* ventilator cycles.

Setting tidal volume

☐ 7. Adjust ventilator settings as follows:

$$V_T = 600 \text{ ml}$$
$$f = 16$$

Inspiratory flow rate = 30

Measure expired V_T with spirometer

V_T = _____

Question: Does this measurement agree with your V_T setting? If not, why not?

Comments:
Calibration of the machine may not be precise.
Calibration of the spirometer may not be precise.
The placement of the spirometer will influence readings.
The spirometer should be beyond the exhalation valve in the expiratory line.
Leaks may exist in the system.

Checking V_T

☐ 8. Turn Autowedge spirometer warning level to 100 to 200 ml less than the V_T

Compare set V_T with Autowedge electronic spirometer reading and your spirometer reading

Set V_T = _____
Reference spirometer V_T = _____
Autowedge electronic spirometer V_T = _____

Question: Do these numbers agree? If not, why not?

Comments:
The Autowedge spirometer (an electrical measuring device) has a variance of ±100 ml.
The V_T setting is much more likely to be accurate than the Autowedge spirometer reading.
Leaks may exist in the system.
Improper calibration of the reference spirometer may influence readings.

Compare set V_T with Autowedge spirometer reading and your spirometer reading.

Set V_T = _____
Reference spirometer V_T = _____
Autowedge mechanical spirometer V_T = _____

Question: Do the numbers agree? If not, why not?

Comments:

The Autowedge mechanical spirometer will vary up to ±100 ml.

Improper seating of the spirometer liner will cause discrepancies.

Improper calibration of the reference spirometer will influence readings.

Setting respiratory rate

☐ 9. Set f at 20

Then verify setting by counting for full minute

f = _____

Question: Does the digital readout of f agree with your count? If not, why not?

Comments:

Several breaths are required for the digital readout to adjust to any new settings.

If the I:E ratio becomes less than 1:1, the respiratory rate will decrease automatically to correct the ratio to 1:1.

Calculation of inspiratory flow

☐ 10. Turn Autowedge warning level to "off" position

Set V$_T$ at 1000 ml

Set f at 10

Calculate inspiratory flow rate with this formula:

V$_E$ × 3 = inspiratory flow rate

Calculated inspiratory flow rate = _____

Set inspiratory flow rate at calculated value

Comments:

This *should* produce an I:E ratio of 1:2.

Each respiratory cycle will last 6 seconds. To achieve an I:E ratio of 1:2, a patient will spend 2 seconds inspiring and 4 seconds exhaling.

You must deliver 1 liter in 2 seconds or 30 liters in 60 seconds to maintain an I:E ratio of 1:2.

This formula may be inadequate for some V$_T$ and f combinations.

Adjust inspiratory flow rate until desired ratio of 1:2 is reached

Required inspiratory flow rate = _____

Measuring I:E ratio

☐ 11. Set inspiratory flow rate at 24 LPM

Set V$_T$ at 600 ml

Set f at 20

Note and record I:E ratio = _____

Correct inspiratory flow rate to achieve I:E ratio of 1:2

I:E ratio = _____
Inspiratory flow = _____

Comments:
The digital readout of the I:E ratio averages the ratios of the previous 5 breaths. Be patient.

If you are not comfortable about manipulating these controls (V_T, IFR, f) practice by changing each one separately.

Fine tuning

☐ 12. Set f at 15
Set V_T at 750 ml
Set inspiratory flow rate at 35 LPM
Verify f with a chronometer

f = _____

Calculate anticipated minute volume

Calculated $\dot{V}_E$ = _____

Measure actual minute volume with spirometer

$\dot{V}_E$ = _____

Question: Is there a difference between calculated and measured $\dot{V}_E$? If so, why? (See comments under tasks 7 and 8.)

Measure V_T with spirometer

V_T = _____

Adjust flow rate to achieve I:E ratio of 1:2

Monitoring maximum inspiratory pressure

☐ 13. Leave settings as in task 12
Watch maximum inspiratory pressure (gauge is marked "airway pressure")

MIP = _____

Set "high inspiratory pressure warning" alarm 10 cm H_2O higher than MIP
Squeeze distal half of test lung while observing pressure gauge and high-inspiratory-pressure alarm

MIP = _____

Comments:
The MIP is the combined resistance in the test lung and the ventilator tubing. The high-inspiratory-warning alarm is usually set 10 cm

H_2O higher than the MIP. However, if the patient's MIP is over 50, the setting should be ordered by the physician.

The inspiratory pressure alarm is an audible alarm that warns you of an increase in pressure. It is *not* a pop-off or pressure relief system.

This warning is inactive during delivery of deep breaths.

☐ 14. Leave settings as in task 12

Note maximum inspiratory pressure

MIP = _____

Set inspiratory pressure relief 20 cm H_2O higher than MIP

Squeeze distal half of test lung while observing pressure gauge and high inspiratory pressure and inspiratory pressure relief alarms

MIP = _____

Comments:

When the pressure reaches the preset limit, inspiration is terminated.

If the deep breath mode is in use, this control should be set at a pressure limit sufficient to deliver the deep breath volume.

The inspiratory pressure relief control is usually set 20 cm H_2O higher than the MIP. However, if the MIP is greater than 50, the setting should be ordered by the physician.

Setting deep breath volumes

☐ 15. Set deep breath volume at 1000 ml

Set deep breath interval at 8 min

Set multiple deep breath at 2

Attach reference spirometer to measure expired volume.

Use "manual deep breath" control to produce a sigh.

Note and record during a deep breath:

Sigh volume = _____
MIP = _____

Calculate:

Sighs/hr = _____

Comments:

Delivery of the proper deep breath volume depends on *not* exceeding the inspiratory pressure relief level.

Maximum inspiratory pressures over 50 cm H_2O may be dangerous. Deep breath volumes may need to be decreased if MIPs are over 50.

The "manual deep breath" control will not work if the interval control is in "off" position.

Verifying F$_{IO_2}$

☐ 16. Set f at 15

Set V$_T$ at 800 ml

Set I:E ratio at 1:2

Insert oxygen analyzer between Y piece of patient circuit and test
  lung

Measure F$_{IO_2}$ at each of the following settings:

F$_{IO_2}$ setting	.21	.4	.6	1.0
Measured value				

Question: Do the measured values agree with the setting? If not, why
  not?

Comments:

Precise agreement requires accurate calibration of the oxygen analyzer. If the variance is within ±5%, the problem may be caused
  by either analyzer or ventilator error. Check the analyzer. (The
  ventilator is usually very stable within ±5%.

If the variance is greater than ±5%, the analyzer must be calibrated. Then recheck the F$_{IO_2}$. (Analyzer accuracy deteriorates with
  time.)

Setting patient triggering effort

☐ 17. Leave settings as in task 16

Turn patient-triggering-effort dial to "min" (if ventilator self-cycles,
  increase setting until ventilator stops self-cycling)

Squeeze test lung and release abruptly while watching airway pressure gauge

Comment: Note that a slight negative pressure is produced. The triggering light comes on, and the ventilator inflates the test lung.

☐ 18. Set patient triggering effort dial at "max"

Squeeze test lung and release abruptly while watching airway pressure gauge

Comment: It should be impossible to trigger a breath with this maneuver. If the control is turned to the "off" position, a breath *cannot* be triggered by the patient.

☐ 19. Adjust ventilator settings as follows:

$$F_{IO_2} = 0.35$$
$$V_T = 800 \text{ ml}$$
$$f = 10$$
$$I:E \text{ ratio} = 1:2$$

Patient triggering effort = "min"

Deep breath volume = 1200 ml

Interval = 6 min

Multiple deep breaths = $\times 2$

Verify settings with spirometer, chronometer, and oxygen analyzer

Observe patient resistance (MIP)

Record all values on ventilator flow sheet

Adjust ventilator settings as follows:

V_T = 600 ml

f = 15

I:E ratio = 1:2

Observe MIP

Verify settings with spirometer, oxygen analyzer, and chronometer

Record all values on ventilator flow sheet

Question: Does the I:E ratio change with changes in V_T? If so, why?

Comment: Respiratory rate, I:E ratio, V_T, and inspiratory flow rate are interrelated. If the volume is decreased but inspiratory flow is kept the same, the inspiratory time will be shortened.

☐ 20. Adjust the ventilator as follows:

$F_{I_{O_2}}$ = 0.7

V_T = 700

f = 20

I:E ratio = 1:2

Deep breath volume = 1200 ml

Interval = 6

Multiple deep breath = $\times 2$

Verify with monitoring equipment

Record on ventilator flow sheet

Change to a smaller size of test lung (or manually occlude distal half of lung now being used)

Observe any changes from what was recorded in previous entry on flow sheet

Comment: Decreasing the lung size (for example, by simulating mucus plugs, or right main stem intubation) increases the MIP.

Use of inflation hold

☐ 21. Leave settings as in task 20

Observe movement of needle on airway pressure gauge; it should reach peak pressure, reverse rapidly, and return to zero

Turn inflation hold dial to 1.0 seconds

Now note pause in needle at end of inspiration

Turn inflation hold dial to zero

Comments:

For therapeutic purposes, this control is used *only* with a physician's order.

This control may be used to measure static pressure.

There probably will be no change in static pressure if you are using a test lung.

☐ 22. Locate "nebulizer off" toggle switch

Comment: This control supplies gas extracted from the tidal volume to the mechanical nebulizer during inspiration when nebulization of drugs is desired.

Setting PEEP

☐ 23. Adjust ventilator settings as follows:

$$F_{I_{O_2}} = 0.6$$
$$V_T = 800 \text{ ml}$$
$$f = 15$$
$$I:E \text{ ratio} = 1:2$$

Patient triggering effort = "max" or "off"

Note MIP

MIP = _____

Set PEEP at 10 cm H_2O by turning PEEP control while watching airway pressure gauge

Note MIP

MIP = _____

Question: What happens to MIP when 10 cm H_2O of PEEP is used?

Comments:

PEEP at any given level may change with changed lung compliance and/or tidal volume. When changing tidal volume, always recheck the level of PEEP delivered.

Because lung compliance can change rapidly in many patients requiring PEEP, this level should be checked at least hourly with all other ventilator settings.

Turn PEEP to zero.

Inspiratory flow taper

☐ 24. Leave settings as in task 20; no action is required

Note inspiratory flow taper control

Comment: This control should be used only with a physician's order. As the control is moved from the "square wave minimum" position counterclockwise, the following happens: after approximately two thirds of the tidal volume has been delivered, the flow diminishes and a longer time is required to deliver the tidal volume. See figure below:

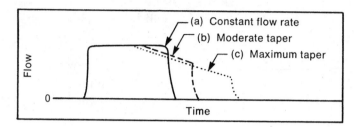

a, constant inspiratory flow rate
b, small amount of flow tapering
c, maximum amount of flow taper

Comment: It is necessary to use a minimum flow rate of 40 LPM when using the inspiratory flow taper control.

Manual breaths

☐ 25. Leave settings as in task 20
Locate "manual inspiration" button
Just *after* an exhaled breath, depress manual inspiration button and hold for several seconds
Note delivery of additional tidal breaths by watching respiratory rate and I:E ratio digital displays

Comment: The response is limited by the flow rate

Locate the "manual deep breath" button; push once
Note the delivery of a deep breath; this breath is cycled in sequence with respiratory rate setting; therefore, it may be delayed by one breath

Comments:

These controls are useful when checking ventilator function or when a patient's ventilatory demands increase momentarily—for example, after turning or suctioning or in response to a painful stimulus.

The manual inspiration button is disabled until the delivery of the deep breath is completed.

Functioning of alarms

☐ 26. Adjust ventilator controls as follows:

$$V_T = 800 \text{ ml}$$
$$f = 15$$
$$I:E \text{ ratio} = 1:2$$

☐ **A. Low inspiratory pressure**

Disconnect test lung

Low inspiratory pressure warning should be triggered at end of next inhalation

Reconnect test lung

Warning resets automatically

Comments:

This alarm is activated if a minimum airway pressure of 8 cm H_2O is not reached by the end of inspiration.

This alarm is self-cancelling.

☐ **B. End-expiratory pressure**

Disconnect exhalation tube from autowedge spirometer and obstruct exhalation to create end-expiratory pressure of 6 cm H_2O or greater

End-expiratory pressure warning should be triggered at end of next exhalation

Spirometer warning also should be triggered

Reconnect exhalation tube and *reset* warnings

Comments:

This alarm activates if the airway pressure is greater than 5 cm H_2O at the end of exhalation.

It is PEEP compensated.

It is self-cancelling.

☐ **C. High inspiratory pressure**

Set high inspiratory pressure warning control 5 cm H_2O lower than maximum pressure indicated on airway pressure gauge

Momentary audible warning should sound, and corresponding lamp should light

Return high inspiratory pressure warning to setting of 100

Comments:

This alarm is PEEP compensated.

It is self-cancelling.

☐ **D. Inspiratory pressure relief**

Set inspiratory pressure relief control 15 cm H_2O lower than pressure registering on airway pressure gauge

Inspiratory pressure relief warnings should be triggered

Tidal volume indicator of Autowedge should show decreased V_T, and spirometer warning signal should sound

Return inspiratory pressure relief setting to 100

Comments:

This alarm is PEEP compensated.

It is self-cancelling.

☐ **E. Short exhalation**

Set V_T at 600 ml

Set f at 30

Set inspiratory flow rate at "min"

Short exhalation warning lamp should light, and respiratory rate displayed should *not* reach 30; I:E ratio of about 1:1 will be maintained

Comments:

This alarm activates if the I:E ratio falls below 1:1.

This alarm is self-cancelling.

The short exhalation warning is a fast response alarm.

The I:E ratio digital readout, however, requires several breaths to equilibrate. Therefore, it is possible to have the short exhalation warning sound while the I:E ratio readout appears acceptable.

☐ **F. Failure to cycle**

Set V_T at 800 ml

Set f at 15

Set I:E ratio of 1:2

Completely obstruct inhalation side of patient tubing system to prevent delivery of tidal volume

Failure-to-cycle warning should be triggered after 13 to 16 seconds

Reset warning

Comment: This alarm activates if over 15 seconds elapse without the delivery of a breath.

☐ **G. Power disconnect**

Disconnect ventilator's electrical power cord from outlet

Power disconnect warning should sound

Plug in cord and reset warning

☐ **H. Low oxygen pressure**

Set oxygen concentration control at 100%

Disconnect oxygen hose from 50 PSI source

Low oxygen pressure warning will sound; spirometer V_T reading should *not* change

Return oxygen concentration control to "off," and reset warning

Reconnect oxygen hose to 50 PSI source

Comment: This alarm activates when the oxygen pressure falls below 10 PSI.

☐ I. **Fan**

Obstruct ventilator's air inlet at fan filter

Audible and visual fan warnings should activate (fan warnings are activated by decreased air flow)

Remove air inlet obstruction

Reset warning

Comment: This alarm activates when the machine is first turned on and at subsequent times if the flow of cooling air becomes insufficient.

Searle ventilation mode controller

☐ 27. Set ventilator controls as follows:

$$V_T = 800 \text{ ml}$$
$$f = 12$$
$$F_{I_{O_2}} = 0.5$$
$$I:E \text{ ratio} = 1:2$$
$$\text{Patient triggering} = \text{"min"}$$

Set mode controller as follows:

$$\text{Apnea warning delay} = 8 \text{ seconds}$$
$$\text{IDV frequency} = 2$$
$$\text{Mode selector} = \text{IDV}$$
$$\text{Power} = \text{"on"}$$

Comment: The apnea warning audible and visual alarm will activate in 8 seconds.

Squeeze and abruptly release the test lung 15 to 20 times per minute to simulate spontaneous breathing.

Comment: These settings and this action will produce a patient-triggered, patient-determined V_T breath followed by a patient-triggered, forced-inspiration V_T breath (V_T will equal what is set on the ventilator). The green "forced inspiration" light will activate.

Stop squeezing test lung

Note:

In 8 seconds, the apnea warning alarm will sound.

The ventilator will begin functioning at your preset values.

Comments:

In this mode, the ventilator is a backup system to the patient's triggering efforts. If the apnea periods exceed preset limits, a warning sounds.

The ratio of IDV to patient-initiated breaths is a constant percentage of breaths, despite changes in respiratory rate.

PEEP may be used with IDV.

☐ 28. Please consult respiratory therapist for use of continuous positive airway pressure (CPAP) controls

☐ 29. Disconnect ventilator from oxygen and electrical sources; secure cords to back of ventilator

Self-guided tour of the MA-1 ventilator

This is one of four similar modules, each of which concentrates on a different ventilator.

This hands-on exercise is designed to familiarize the student with the ventilator controls, displays, and mechanics.

Students usually work in pairs. Each pair proceeds at its own pace. An instructor is on call nearby.

One instructor can supervise three pairs.

Objectives The student will establish V_T, f, $I:E$ ratio, sigh volume, frequency of sigh, FI_{O_2}, and level of patient triggering effort and will enable and disable alarms at a variety of settings.

The student will verify settings by using a spirometer and an oxygen analyzer.

The student will record measurements on a ventilator flow sheet.

Equipment required
1. MA-1 ventilator
2. Rubber test lung*
3. Wright or Draeger spirometer
4. Oxygen analyzer
5. Ventilator flow sheet
6. Patient circuit
7. Chronometer

Skills required
1. Ability to use spirometer
2. Ability to use oxygen analyzer
3. Ability to measure $I:E$ ratio

TO INSTRUCTORS: The ventilator should have all controls in "off" or disabled positions and volumes at zero, *except* that pressure or volume alarms or pop-offs should be operative at maximum levels.

The ventilator should not be plugged in to an electrical outlet or connected to an oxygen source.

Tasks

☐ 1. Review locations of the following:

Indication lights
    Assist
    Pressure
    Ratio

*The test lung should have a reasonably stiff compliance, and the compliance band should be intact.

Sigh
Oxygen
Controls
Sensitivity
Peak flow
Power
Nebulizer
Sigh volume
Normal pressure limit
Normal volume
Rate
Oxygen percentage
Sighs—per hour and multiple
Manual—normal
Manual—sigh
Sigh pressure limit
Expiratory resistance

☐ 2. Turn power switch off
☐ 3. Plug power cord into grounded 110-volt AC outlet
☐ 4. Connect oxygen high pressure hose directly to 50 PSI oxygen source
☐ 5. Connect test lung to Y piece of patient circuit
☐ 6. Turn power switch on

Setting tidal volume

☐ 7. Adjust ventilator settings as follows:

$$V_T = 600 \text{ ml}$$
$$f = 16$$
Peak flow rate = 30 LPM

Measure expired V_T with spirometer

$V_T =$ _____

Question: Does this measurement agree with your V_T setting? If not, why?

Comments:
Calibration of the machine may not be precise.
Calibration of the spirometer may not be precise.
Placement of the spirometer may influence readings.
The spirometer should be beyond the exhalation valve in the expiratory line.
Leaks may exist in the system.
The ventilator adds 50 ml to V_T to compensate for tubing compliance.

174

Setting respiratory rate

☐ 8. Set f at 20

Measure f by counting for full minute

f = _____

Calculating peak flow

☐ 9. Adjust ventilator settings as follows:

V_T = 1000 ml
f = 10

Calculate peak flow by this formula:
$\dot{V}_E \times 3$ = Peak flow

Calculated peak flow = _____

Set peak flow at calculated value

Comments:
This should produce an I:E ratio of 1:2.

If f is 10 and tidal volume is 1000 ml, then each respiratory cycle will
be 6 seconds in length. To achieve an I:E ratio of 1:2, the patient
should spend 2 seconds in inspiration and 4 seconds in exhalation.

You must deliver 1 liter in 2 seconds or 30 liters in 60 seconds to
maintain an I:E ratio of 1:2.

This flow is limited by high airway pressures and in certain instances
may need to be set somewhat higher.

If the ratio achieved is less than 1:1, the ratio indicator light and an
audible signal will be activated.

Measure I:E ratio

I:E ratio = _____

Correct peak flow to achieve ratio of 1:2

Peak flow at I:E ratio of 1:2 = _____

Setting peak flow

☐ 10. Set V_T at 600 ml

Set f at 12

Calculate and set peak flow

Calculated peak flow = _____

Determine I:E ratio

I:E ratio = _____

Correct peak flow to achieve I:E ratio of 1:2

Peak flow = _____

Comment: If you are not comfortable manipulating these controls
(V_T, IFR, f), practice by changing each one separately.

Setting controls

☐ 11. Set V_T at 900 ml
Set f at 15
Calculate and set peak flow
Verify V_T with spirometer

V_T = _____

Verify f with chronometer

f = _____

Calculate anticipated $\dot{V}_E$

Anticipated $\dot{V}_E$ = _____

Measure actual $\dot{V}_E$ with a spirometer

$\dot{V}_E$ = _____

Determine I:E ratio

I:E ratio = _____

Adjust peak flow to achieve I:E ratio of 1:2

Monitoring maximum inspiratory pressure

☐ 12. Leave settings as in task 11
Note maximum inspiratory pressure (gauge is marked "system pressure")

MIP = _____

Kink inspiratory tubing sharply while observing pressure gauge

MIP = _____

Comments:
Inspiration will cease when the pressure set by the normal pressure limit is reached.
The MIP is caused by the combined resistance in the test lung and the ventilator tubing. The normal pressure limit is usually set about 15 cm H_2O higher than the actual MIP. However, if the patient's MIP is over 50, the limit should be ordered by a physician.

Setting sigh volume and pressure limits

☐ 13. Set sigh volume at 1200 ml
Set sighs per hour at 6 × 2
Attach spirometer to measure expired volumes
Use "manual—sigh" control to produce a sigh

V_{sigh} = _____

Note MIP

MIP = _____

Set sigh pressure limit 10 cm H_2O higher than sigh volume MIP

Kink inspiratory line sharply while observing pressure gauge

MIP = _____

Comments:

Inspiration will cease when the pressure limit is reached.

If the sigh volume produces a maximum inspiratory pressure of 40 cm H_2O and the sigh pressure limit is set at 30 cm H_2O, the preset sigh volume will *not* be delivered in full.

Always set sigh pressure limit about 10 to 15 cm H_2O higher than the level normally produced by the sigh volume.

Maximum inspiratory pressures over 50 cm H_2O may be dangerous.

Sigh volumes may need to be decreased if MIPs over 50 are generated.

Verifying F_{IO_2}

☐ 14. Insert oxygen analyzer between Y piece of patient circuit and test lung

Measure F_{IO_2} at each of the following settings:

F_{IO_2} setting	.21	.4	.6	1.0
Measured value				

Question: Do the measured values agree with the settings?

Comments:

Precise agreement requires accurate calibration of the oxygen analyzer. If the variance is within ±5%, the problem may be caused by either analyzer or ventilator error. Check the analyzer. (The ventilator is usually very stable within ±5%.)

If the variance is greater than ±5%, the analyzer must be recalibrated. Then recheck the F_{IO_2}. (Analyzer accuracy deteriorates with time.)

Patience is required. The response time of the ventilator may be as long as 60 seconds.

Altering settings

☐ 15. Adjust ventilator settings as follows:

$$V_T = 800 \text{ ml}$$
$$F_{IO_2} = .35$$
$$I:E \text{ ratio} = 1:2$$
$$f = 12$$
$$\text{Sigh volume} = 1500 \text{ ml}$$
$$\text{Sighs per hour} = 6$$
$$\text{Multi-sigh} = \times 2$$

Verify settings with your spirometer, chronometer, and oxygen analyzer

Record all values on ventilator flow sheet

Question: Does the I : E ratio change with changes in V_T?

Comment: Respiratory rate, I : E ratio, V_T, and inspiratory flow rate are interrelated. If the volume is decreased but inspiratory flow is kept the same, the inspiratory time will be shortened.

Simulating patient changes

☐ 16. Adjust ventilator settings as follows:

$$V_T = 700 \text{ ml}$$
$$F_{I_{O_2}} = 0.7$$
$$f = 10$$
$$\text{I : E ratio} = 1 : 2$$
$$\text{Sigh volume} = 1200 \text{ ml}$$
$$\text{Sighs per hour} = 8$$
$$\text{Multi-sigh} = \times 3$$

Verify settings with monitoring equipment

Record on ventilator flow sheet

Change to smaller size of test lung (or manually occlude distal half of lung now being used)

Observe any changes from what was recorded in previous entry

Comment: Decreasing the lung size (for example, by simulating mucus plugs or right main stem intubation) increases the MIP.

Setting sensitivity

☐ 17. Set sensitivity dial at "min" (if ventilator self-cycles, increase setting until ventilator stops self-cycling)

Squeeze and abruptly release test lung while watching MIP

Comments:

Note that a slight negative pressure is produced.

The triggering light comes on, and the ventilator inflates the test lung.

With the setting in this position, it is easy for the patient to initiate breaths.

☐ 18. Set sensitivity dial at "max"

Squeeze and abruptly release test lung while watching MIP

Comments:

It should be impossible to trigger a breath during this maneuver.

With the setting in this position, it is impossible for the patient to "turn on" the ventilator.

Functioning of alarms

☐ 19. Disconnect a tube in inspiratory line
Note alarm
Disable alarm
Reconnect tube
Reset alarm

Comment: Only the spirometer alarm will indicate disconnection from the patient, leaks, or failure of the machine to cycle.

☐ 20. If you cannot answer questions or do not feel comfortable manipulating controls, seek help from instructor

☐ 21. Turn power off
Disconnect high pressure oxygen hose from 50 PSI source and secure to back of ventilator
Disconnect power cord and secure to back of ventilator

Ventilator application

Overview These are team exercises in decision-making. They require the team to adjust simulated patient-ventilator systems in response to key data. The decision-making process is structured in accordance with the various chapters of this book.

Instructor Any exceptionally knowledgeable member of the team may act as the instructor.

Target group These exercises are intended for MDs, RNs, and RTs who are responsible for patients attached to ventilators. The exercises are aimed at beginners or persons who may not be involved regularly in the care of ventilator patients.

Objectives At the end of these exercises, a student will be able to use this book to make the following decisions correctly when provided with the necessary data:

1. Determine whether patient satisfies criteria for intubation and mechanical ventilation (Chapter 2)
2. Specify treatment goals in terms of Pa_{O_2}, Pa_{CO_2}, and pH (Chapter 7)
3. Specify whether volume-cycled ventilator would be preferred to pressure-cycled ventilator and why (Chapter 5)
4. Specify initial settings that should be established on simulated patient system before connecting ventilator to real patient (Chapter 7)
5. Record on ventilator flow sheet blood gas data in some column or row as related ventilator data, that is, the conditions that influenced the blood gases (Chapter 15)
6. Use the following equation (Chapter 12) to approximate more desirable V_T', f' and/or Pa_{CO_2}':

$$V_T \cdot f \cdot Pa_{CO_2} = V_T' \cdot f' \cdot Pa_{CO_2}'$$

7. Adjust FI_{O_2} downward from 1.0 in accordance with guidelines (Chapter 11)
8. Determine whether patient satisfies criteria for use of PEEP (Chapter 21)
9. Use decision guide (algorithm) to carry out "PEEP study" and to select "best PEEP" (Chapter 21)

10. Select candidates for "weaning challenge" of brief trial session on T piece (Chapter 22)
11. Indicate whether patient has "passed" or "failed" "weaning challenge" (Chapter 22)

Time frame The situations can be completed in 3 to 4 sessions of 60 to 90 minutes each.

Setting An appropriate setting is a vacant intensive care room or other space that provides the following:

Space for team and ventilator

110-volt AC outlet

50 PSI oxygen source

Space where instructor can withdraw from the team yet observe and be available

Materials
1. Ventilator of type(s) to be used by students in their own hospitals
2. Oxygen blender (if not built into ventilator)
3. Spirometer
4. Simulated patient (rubber test lung, mannikin, or bellows)*
5. Situations 1, 2, 3, 4, and 5
6. Blood gas requisition form (Copies of this form should be available for each of the exercises.)
7. Blood gas slide rule(s)
8. Hand calculator(s) or slide rule(s)
9. Clip boards
10. Copies of this book

Pretest No pretest is required. Students who have completed successfully the previous exercises in this book will be qualified for these exercises.

Post-test No post-test is required. The exercises are structured in a manner that permits the instructor to make unobstrusive comparison of students' speed, skill, and accuracy.

*These exercises are adapted for use with the "lung simulator," which is manufactured for The Manley Lung Ventilator Performance Analyser Company by Medical Developments Ltd., Beaconsfield, Bucks, England (patent applied for). This device can accept VTs of up to 1000 ml. Two lung simulators operating in parallel can be used to simulate the breathing of patients who weigh more than 45 kg. These exercises are also adaptable for use with a rubber test lung.

Ventilator application situation 1

To instructors   A typical student team consists of an MD, an RN, and an RT.

1. Briefly explain the purpose of the sessions and the exercises.
2. Explain that you will provide simulated blood gas test results whenever the team wants these data but that requests must be submitted in writing on the form that is provided.
3. Distribute Situation 1, tasks 1 to 6, and the blood gas test requisition forms. Instruct the team members to check with you after each task. Call attention to this book, and explain that all decisions will be arbitrated on the material in the book.
4. Withdraw from the team slightly, and let the team members reach concensus on each decision. When you are consulted, ask the team's reasons for each of its recommendations. Point out those recommendations that are not consistent with the book. (Avoid implications of "right" and "wrong." Instead, point out what is recommended and in accordance with the rationale.)
5. Task 6 requires the team to obtain blood gas test results after the patient has been attached to the ventilator for 20 minutes. Feed back results that are not close enough to the team's stated goals. This will simulate the initial trial-and-error process that is usually required to achieve the desired blood gas levels with a patient-ventilator system. Have the team calculate a new f' and/or V_T' at least twice. Insist that all data be entered in the flow sheet promptly as they are obtained.
6. When the team has completed tasks 1 to 6, distribute tasks 7 and 8, which are concerned with determining the patient's readiness for weaning. The team is required to decide in late afternoon whether to try the T piece the next morning or to wait until the patient is in better shape. The decision should be arbitrated by referring to the appropriate chapter of the book. In these tasks, the team is not required to simulate any adjustments on the ventilator.
7. When the team has completed tasks 7 and 8, distribute tasks 9 and 10, in which the results of a hypothetical 20-minute trial session with the T piece are provided. The team is required to decide whether the patient has "passed" or "failed" the challenge. The team is also required to make recommendations about the next steps in weaning the patient. Tasks 9 and 10 do not require the team to simulate the T piece setup or standby settings.

Blood gas analysis requisitions

You will need blood gas data to complete some tasks in the following exercises. When you need such data, fill out one of the requisitions provided below, and submit it to the instructor.

Blood gas analysis requisition form

Situation No. _____
Time _____ hrs.
$\dot{V}_E$ _____ LPM
$F_{I_{O_2}}$ _____

BE _____
pH _____
Pa_{CO_2} _____
Pa_{O_2} _____

Blood gas analysis requisition form

Situation No. _____
Time _____ hrs.
$\dot{V}_E$ _____ LPM
$F_{I_{O_2}}$ _____

BE _____
pH _____
Pa_{CO_2} _____
Pa_{O_2} _____

Blood gas analysis requisition form

Situation No. _____
Time _____ hrs.
$\dot{V}_E$ _____ LPM
$F_{I_{O_2}}$ _____

BE _____
pH _____
Pa_{CO_2} _____
Pa_{O_2} _____

Blood gas analysis requisition form

Situation No. _____
Time _____ hrs.
$\dot{V}_E$ _____ LPM
$F_{I_{O_2}}$ _____

BE _____
pH _____
Pa_{CO_2} _____
Pa_{O_2} _____

Blood gas analysis requisition form

Situation No. _____
Time _____ hrs.
$\dot{V}_E$ _____ LPM
$F_{I_{O_2}}$ _____

BE _____
pH _____
Pa_{CO_2} _____
Pa_{O_2} _____

Blood gas analysis requisition form

Situation No. _____
Time _____ hrs.
$\dot{V}_E$ _____ LPM
$F_{I_{O_2}}$ _____

BE _____
pH _____
Pa_{CO_2} _____
Pa_{O_2} _____

Blood gas analysis requisition form

Situation No. _____
Time _____ hrs.
$\dot{V}_E$ _____ LPM
$F_{I_{O_2}}$ _____

BE _____
pH _____
Pa_{CO_2} _____
Pa_{O_2} _____

Blood gas analysis requisition form

Situation No. _____
Time _____ hrs.
$\dot{V}_E$ _____ LPM
$F_{I_{O_2}}$ _____

BE _____
pH _____
Pa_{CO_2} _____
Pa_{O_2} _____

Situation 1　Your patient is a 25-year-old female who was healthy until today when she took an overdose of barbiturates. Her respiratory rate is 6 BPM. Her lungs seem clear. Her weight is 50 kg. Her initial blood gas levels (while breathing room air) are as follows: Pa_{O_2} = 65, Pa_{CO_2} = 65, pH = 7.24, BE = -4, HCO_3 = 23.

Task 1

Intubation and mechanical ventilation are indicated because:

☐ Pa_{O_2} cannot be maintained above 50 mm Hg by increasing $F_{I_{O_2}}$
☐ Pa_{CO_2} has risen above 50 mm Hg and forced pH below 7.25
☐ Effective ventilation has become inefficient and/or exhausting (f greater than 30 or VC less than 20 ml/kg)

**Instructor sign off
(Enter time)**

☐ Other (specify) _____

_____

Task 2

Specify your treatment goals in terms of Pa_{O_2}, and Pa_{CO_2}, and pH:

1. Keep Pa_{O_2} at _____
2. Keep Pa_{CO_2} at _____ and pH at _____

Task 3

Specify the type of ventilator preferred in this case:

☐ Pressure-cycled
☐ Volume-cycled

Task 4

Specify the initial ventilator settings that you would use:

V_T	f	I:E	Flow rate	$F_{I_{O_2}}$	Sensitivity	Sigh

Task 5

Initiate ventilation in accordance with the above settings. (Use a bag or a bellows to simulate the patient's lungs.) Have your instructor check when you are ready.

Task 6

Assume that you have ventilated the patient at your initial settings for 20 minutes. Evaluate your settings and adjust as necessary.

Blood gas test results must be obtained from the laboratory.

Requisitions must be marked with the time of the sample and with $F_{I_{O_2}}$, and $\dot{V}E$ prevailing at that time.

In making your adjustments, you may assume the following relationship between old and new values:

$$V_T \cdot f \cdot Pa_{CO_2} = V_T' \cdot f' \cdot Pa_{CO_2}'$$

Enter all data on the flow sheet below.
When you have achieved your goals, check with your instructor.

Date/hour:	Base-line						
F_{IO_2}							
Pa_{O_2}							
BE/HCO_3							
pH							
Pa_{CO_2}							
$\dot{V}_E$	—						
V_T	—						
f							
I:E ratio	—						
IFR	—						
Control/assist	—						
MIP	—						
Dynamic compliance	—						
Static pressure	—						
Static compliance	—						

Situation 1— cont'd

It is 1700 hours (5 PM) on the second hospital day. The patient is alert again. Chest x-ray film is clear. T = 37.5, HR = 90, BP = 120/70.

The patient is triggering ventilator at the rate of 10 BPM. V_T = 500 ml, FVC = 2000 ml. Peak pressure is 30 cm H_2O. The patient can generate an inspiratory force of −50 cm H_2O. Blood gas levels (F_{IO_2} = 0.21) are: Pa_{O_2} = 80, Pa_{CO_2} = 38.

Task 7

Do you believe that this patient is ready for weaning?

☐ Yes
☐ No (give reason) _____

Task 8

If you believe that this patient is ready for weaning, write the orders for the

next step(s): _____

_____

_____

_____

_____

**Situation 1—
cont'd**

At 0800 (8 AM) the next day the patient's condition is still satisfactory, and weaning is begun. She is given a trial session with a T piece with an F_{IO_2} of 0.21. The patient is monitored over the next 20 minutes and then returned to the ventilator (original settings are resumed).

Observations

	Still on "assist"	On T-piece				Back on "assist"
Time	0800	0805	0810	0815	0820	0825
f	10	12	14	17	20	12
BP	120/70	125/75	125/75	130/50	140/85	125/75
PR	100	95	100	105	110	100
PVCs	0	0	0	0	0	0
Accessory muscles	0	0	0	0	0	0
Distress	0	0	0	0	0	0
V_T	600	300	300	290	295	600
VC	2000				1900	
Pa_{O_2} (0.21)	80				75	
Pa_{CO_2}	38				41	
pH	7.38				7.36	

Task 9

Did the patient pass the challenge?

☐ Yes
☐ No, the patient failed at _____ hours.

Task 10

Write your orders for the next step: _____

_____

Ventilator application situation 2

To instructors A typical student team consists of an MD, an RN, and an RT.

1. Briefly explain the purpose of the sessions and the exercises.
2. Explain that you will provide simulated blood gas test results whenever the team wants these data but that requests must be submitted in writing on the form that is provided.
3. Distribute Situation 2, tasks 1 to 6, and the blood gas test requisition forms. Instruct the team members to check with you after each task. Call attention to this book, and explain that all decisions will be arbitrated on the material in the book.
4. Withdraw from the team slightly, and let the team members reach consensus on each decision. When you are consulted, ask the team's reasons for each of its recommendations. Point out those recommendations that are not consistent with the book. (Avoid implications of "right" and "wrong." Instead point out what is recommended and in accordance with the rationale.)
5. Task 6 requires the team to obtain blood gas test results after the patient has been attached to the ventilator for 20 minutes. Feed back results that are not close enough to the team's stated goals. This will simulate the initial trial-and-error process that is usually required to achieve the desired blood gas levels with a patient-ventilator system. Have the team calculate a new f' and/or V_T' at least twice. Insist that all data be entered in the flow sheet promptly as they are obtained.
6. When the team has completed tasks 1 to 6, distribute tasks 7 and 8, which are concerned with determining the patient's readiness for weaning. The team is required to decide in late afternoon whether to try the T piece the next morning or to wait until the patient is in better shape. The decision should be arbitrated by referring to the appropriate chapter of the book. In these tasks, the team is not required to simulate any adjustments on the ventilator.
7. When the team has completed tasks 7 and 8, distribute tasks 9 and 10, in which the results of a hypothetical 20-minute trial session with the T piece are provided. The team is required to decide whether the patient has "passed" or "failed" the challenge. The team is also required to make recommendations about the next steps in weaning the patient. Tasks 9 and 10 do not require the team to simulate T piece setup or standby settings.

Situation 2   Your patient is a 55-year-old male with COPD. He seemed compensated two weeks ago when you saw him last (Pa_{O_2} = 57, Pa_{CO_2} = 54, pH = 7.38, BE = +5, HCO_3 = 31). Two days ago, he developed influenza. Today he was admitted in stupor with f = 18. His initial blood gas levels while breathing O_2 by mask ($F_{I_{O_2}}$ = 0.28) showed: Pa_{O_2} = 45, Pa_{CO_2} = 80, pH = 7.24, BE = +3, HCO_3 = 33. He weighs 60 kg.

Task 1

Intubation and mechanical ventilation are indicated because:

☐ Pa_{O_2} cannot be maintained above 50 by increasing $F_{I_{O_2}}$
☐ Pa_{CO_2} has risen above 50 and forced pH below 7.25
☐ Effective ventilation has become inefficient and/or exhausting (f greater than 30 or VC less than 20 ml/kg)
☐ Other (specify) _____

_____

Task 2

Specify your treatment goals in terms of Pa_{O_2}, Pa_{CO_2}, and pH:

1. Keep Pa_{O_2} at ___ 70 mm Hg ___
2. Keep Pa_{CO_2} at ___ 40 ___ and pH at ___ 7.35 ___

Task 3

Specify the type of ventilator preferred in this case:

☐ Pressure-cycled
☑ Volume-cycled

Task 4

Specify the initial ventilator settings that you would use:

V_T	f	I : E	Flow rate	$F_{I_{O_2}}$	Sensitivity	Sigh
600	10	1:2	18	.50		-2

Task 5

Initiate ventilation in accordance with the above settings. (Use a bag or a bellows to simulate the patient's lungs.) Have your instructor check when you are ready.

Task 6

Assume that you have ventilated the patient at your initial settings for 20 minutes. Evaluate your settings and adjust as necessary.

Blood gas results must be obtained from the laboratory.

Requisitions must be marked with the time of the sample and with $F_{I_{O_2}}$, and $\dot{V}E$ prevailing at that time.

In making your adjustments, you may assume the following relationship between old and new values:

$$V_T \cdot f \cdot Pa_{CO_2} = V_T' \cdot f' \cdot Pa_{CO_2}'$$

Enter all data on the flow sheet below.

When you have achieved your goals, check with your instructor.

Date/hour:	Base-line						
F_{IO_2}	25	.45	.35	.35			
Pa_{O_2}	45	193	143	120			
BE/HCO_3	+5	33	33	33			
pH	7.24	7.60	7.60	7.36			
Pa_{CO_2}	80	35	35	61			
$\dot{V}_E$	—	6.2					
V_T	—	600	600	400			
f	18	10	10	10			
I:E ratio	—	1:2	1:2				
IFR	—	18	18				
Control/assist	—	10	10				
MIP	—						
Dynamic compliance	—						
Static pressure	—						
Static compliance	—						

Situation 2—cont'd

It is 1700 hours (5 PM) on the third hospital day. The patient is alert again. T = 37, HR = 100, BP = 160/90. The patient has some expiratory wheezes throughout both lungs. Chest x-ray film is clear.

The patient is triggering the ventilator at 10 BPM. V_T = 900 ml, FVC = 600 ml. Peak pressure is 45 cm H_2O. Patient is able to generate an inspiratory force of 25 cm H_2O. On F_{IO_2} of 0.35, Pa_{O_2} = 65, Pa_{CO_2} = 40, pH = 7.53.

Task 7

Do you believe that this patient is ready for weaning?

☑ Yes

☐ No (give reason) _____

_____

Task 8

If you believe that this patient is ready for weaning, write the orders for the

next step(s): _____

_____

_____

Situation 2— cont'd

At 0800 (8 AM) the next day, the patient's condition is improved. Wheezing has decreased in response to bronchodilators. Peak pressure has come down to 30 cm H_2O. The patient is triggering the ventilator at 10 BPM. With an F_{IO_2} of 0.35, V_T = 600 ml, Pa_{O_2} = 65, Pa_{CO_2} = 57, pH = 7.37. The patient is given a trial session with the T piece with an F_{IO_2} of 0.35 for 20 minutes and then returned to the ventilator.

Observations

	Still on "assist"	On T-piece				Back on "assist"
Time	0800	0805	0810	0815	0820	0825
f	10	17	17	17	17	10
BP	160/90	170/100	170/100	170/96	180/98	160/80
PR	100	115	115	115	120	105
PVCs	0	0	0	0	2/min	0
Accessory muscles	0	0	0	0	0	0
Distress	0	0	0	0	0	0
V_T	600	300	300	250	250	600
VC	600				550	
Pa_{O_2} on 35%	65				55	
Pa_{CO_2}	55				65	
pH	7.38				7.26	

Task 9

Did the patient pass the challenge?

☐ Yes

☐ No, the patient failed at _____ hours.

Task 10

Write your orders for the next step: _____

_____

_____

Ventilator application situation 3

To instructors A typical student team consists of an MD, an RN, and an RT. Situation 3 is designed to simulate the problems of "shock lung."

1. Briefly explain the purpose of the sessions and the exercises.
2. Explain that you will provide simulated blood gas test results whenever the team wants these data but that requests must be submitted in writing on the form that is provided.
3. Distribute Situation 3, tasks 1 to 6, and the blood gas test requisition forms. Instruct the team members to check with you after each task. Call attention to this book, and explain that all decisions will be arbitrated on the material in the book.
4. Withdraw from the team slightly, and let the team members reach consensus on each decision. When you are consulted, ask the team's reasons for each of its recommendations. Point out those recommendations that are not consistent with the book. Avoid implications of "right" and "wrong." Instead, point out what is recommended and in accordance with the rationale.
5. Task 6 requires the team to obtain blood gas test results after the patient has been attached to the ventilator for 20 minutes. Feed back results that lead in the direction of the situation described in tasks 7 and 8. (Pa_{O_2} should remain low, and a slight metabolic acidosis should be developing.) Have the team calculate a new f' and/or V_T' at least twice. Insist that all data be entered in the flow sheet promptly as they are obtained.
6. When the team has completed tasks 1 to 6, distribute tasks 7 and 8, which require the team to make a decision about the desirability of applying PEEP. The team should consult the first page of the PEEP algorithm (p. 119). The team is required to write orders initiating a PEEP study but is not required to simulate any adjustments on the ventilator.
7. Tasks 9 to 19 are exercises in decision making and require no manipulation of the ventilator. In working them, the team should consult the second page of the PEEP algorithm (p. 120).

   Distribute task 9. When it is complete, proceed to tasks 10 and 11. These tasks lead the team through an uncomplicated PEEP study.

   Tasks 12 to 19 provide examples of unacceptable consequences of various levels of PEEP. Students are required to recognize these consequences and to retreat to a lower level of PEEP.

   Distribute each exercise as the previous one is completed.
8. When the team has completed tasks 9 to 19, distribute tasks 20 and 21. These tasks return the patient to the team as he recovers. The team should consult the section "Adjusting PEEP" (p. 127).
9. After the team has completed tasks 20 and 21, distribute tasks 22 and 23, which require the team to determine the patient's readiness for weaning. The team has to decide whether to try the T piece the next morning or to wait until the patient is in better shape.

10. After the team has completd tasks 22 and 23, distribute tasks 24 and 25, in which the results of a hypothetical 20-minute trial session with the T piece are provided. The team is required to decide whether the patient has "passed" or "failed" the challenge. The team is also required to make recommendations after the next steps in weaning the patient. Tasks 24 and 25 do not require the team to stimulate T piece setup or standby settings.

Situation 3 Your patient is a 37-year-old male jockey. He was injured while racing yesterday. Both femurs are fractured, and at least two ribs are broken. He appears to have "shock lung." His f = 55. He is breathing 40% O_2 by Venti-Mask. His blood gas levels are: Pa_{O_2} = 45, Pa_{CO_2} = 37, pH = 7.38, BE = −2, HCO_3 = 21. He weighs 45 kg. *fat embolus, ARDS*

Task 1

Intubation and mechanical ventilation are indicated because:

☐ Pa_{O_2} cannot be maintained above 50 by increasing F_{IO_2}
☐ Pa_{CO_2} has risen above 50 and forced pH below 7.25
☐ Effective ventilation has become inefficient and/or exhausting (f greater than 30 or VC less than 20 ml/kg)

**Instructor sign off
(Enter time)**

☐ Other (specify) _____

_____

Task 2

Specify your treatment goals in terms of Pa_{O_2}, Pa_{CO_2}, and pH:

1. Keep Pa_{O_2} at _____
2. Keep Pa_{CO_2} at _____ and pH at _____

Task 3

Specify the type of ventilator preferred in this case:

☐ Pressure-cycled
☐ Volume-cycled

Task 4

Specify the initial ventilator settings that you would use:

V_T	f	I : E	Flow rate	F_{IO_2}	Sensitivity	Sigh
700	12	1:2				

Task 5

Initiate ventilation in accordance with the above settings. (Use a bag or a bellows to simulate the patient's lungs.) Have your instructor check when you are ready.

Task 6

Assume that you have ventilated the patient at your initial settings for 20 minutes. Evaluate your settings and adjust as necessary.

Blood gas test results must be obtained from the laboratory.

Requisitions must be marked with the time of the sample and with F_{IO_2}, and $\dot{V}E$ prevailing at that time.

In making your adjustments, you may assume the following relationship between old and new values:

$$V_T \cdot f \cdot Pa_{CO_2} = V_T' \cdot f' \cdot Pa_{CO_2}'$$

Enter all data on the flow sheet below.

When you have achieved your goals, check with your instructor.

Instructor sign off

Observations

Date/hour:	Base-line						
$F_{I_{O_2}}$							
Pa_{O_2}							
BE/HCO_3							
pH							
Pa_{CO_2}							
$\dot{V}_E$	—						
V_T	—						
f							
I : E ratio	—						
IFR	—						
Control/assist	—						
MIP	—						
Dynamic compliance	—						
Static pressure	—						
Static compliance	—						

Situation 3—cont'd

The patient has been attached to the ventilator two days. $Pa_{O_2} = 50$ while breathing 80% O_2. $Pa_{CO_2} = 32$, pH = 7.35. The patient is being ventilated at f = 12, $V_T = 700$ ml. Blood pressure is holding at 110/70 with no respiratory variation. PAW is 10 to 12 mm Hg.

Task 7

Is PEEP justified at this point?

☐ Yes

☐ No (give reason) _____

_____

Task 8

If PEEP is indicated, write orders initiating the PEEP study: _____

_____

_____

A PEEP study is initiated. The following baseline data are obtained:

Observations

	PEEP steps				
PEEP (cm H_2O)	0	5	10	15	0
Time started	1200	1215			
MIP (cm H_2O)	34	37			
Static pressure	31	32			
V_T	700	700			
Systolic (respiratory swing) insp.	110	105			
exp.	115	110			
A-$V_{D_{O_2}}$ (ml O_2/100 ml blood)	4.5				
Pa_{O_2} (FI_{O_2} = 1.0)	60				
Pa_{CO_2}	37				

Task 9

Should the PEEP study be continued?

☑ Yes; obtain blood gas studies.

☐ No; using 5 cm PEEP has the following unacceptable consequences:

Increase to 10 cm H_2O

_____

_____

Instructor sign off

The PEEP study is continued. Additional measurements are carried out on 5 cm H_2O PEEP.

Observations

	PEEP steps				
PEEP (cm H_2O)	0	5	10	15	0
Time started	1200	1215			
MIP (cm H_2O)	34	37			
Static pressure	31	32			
V_T	700	700			
Systolic (respiratory swing) insp.	110	105			
exp.	115	110			
A-$V_{D_{O_2}}$ (ml O_2/100 ml blood)	4.5	4.7			
Pa_{O_2} (FI_{O_2} = 1.0)	60	70			
Pa_{CO_2}	37	38			

Task 10

Should the PEEP study be continued?

☐ Yes; try 10 cm H_2O PEEP.

☐ No; using 5 cm H_2O PEEP has the following unacceptable consequences:

_____

_____

_____

_____

Situation 3—cont'd

The PEEP study is completed without any problems. The following data are available:

Observations

		PEEP steps			
PEEP (cm H_2O)	0	5	10	15	0
Time started	1200	1215	1230	1245	1300
MIP (cm H_2O)	34	37	41	46	32
Static pressure	31	32	34	38	30
V_T	700	700	700	700	700
Systolic insp. (respiratory swing)	110	105	100	95	115
exp.	115	110	105	110	110
A-$V_{D_{O_2}}$ (ml O_2/100 ml blood)	4.5	4.7	4.8	5.2	4.3
Pa_{O_2} ($F_{I_{O_2}} = 1.0$)	60	70	110	80	65
Pa_{CO_2}	37	38	38	40	36

Task 11

What should the team do now ? _____

_____

_____

_____

_____

Situation 3—
cont'd

Observations

Assume that the PEEP study proceeded as indicated in the flow sheet below:

	PEEP steps				
PEEP (cm H_2O)	0	5	10	15	0
Time started	1200	1215	1230		
MIP (cm H_2O)	34	37	48		
Static pressure	31	32	32		
V_T	700	700	700		
Systolic insp. (respiratory swing) exp.	110 115	105 110	105 110		
A-$V_{D_{O_2}}$ (ml O_2/100 ml blood)	4.5	4.7			
Pa_{O_2} (FI_{O_2} = 1.0)	60	70			
Pa_{CO_2}	37	38			

Task 12

Should the PEEP study be continued?

☐ Yes; obtain blood gas studies.
☐ No; using 10 cm H_2O PEEP has the following unacceptable consequences: _____

Instructor sign off

_____

_____

_____

Situation 3—
cont'd

Observations

Assume that the PEEP study proceeded as indicated in the flow sheet below:

	PEEP steps				
PEEP (cm H_2O)	0	5	10	15	0
Time started	1200	1215	1230		
MIP (cm H_2O)	34	37	52		
Static pressure	31	32	38		
V_T	700	700	700		
Systolic insp. (respiratory swing) exp.	110 115	105 110	100 110		
A-$V_{D_{O_2}}$ (ml O_2/100 ml blood)	4.5	4.7			
Pa_{O_2} (FI_{O_2} = 1.0)	60	70			
Pa_{CO_2}	37	37			

Task 13

What should the team do at this point? _____

_____

_____

_____

_____

Situation 3—cont'd

Assume that the PEEP study proceeded as indicated in the flow sheet below:

Observations

		PEEP steps			
PEEP (cm H_2O)		0	5	10	15	0
Time started		1200	1215	1230		
MIP (cm H_2O)		34	37	46		
Static pressure		31	32	44		
V_T		700	700	700		
Systolic (respiratory swing)	insp.	110	105	98		
	exp.	115	110	100		
A-$V_{D_{O_2}}$ (ml O_2/100 ml blood)		4.5	4.7			
Pa_{O_2} ($Fi_{O_2} = 1.0$)		60	70			
Pa_{CO_2}		37	37			

Task 14

What should the team do at this point? _____

_____

_____

_____

_____

Assume that the PEEP study proceeded as indicated in the flow sheet below:

Observations

	PEEP steps				
PEEP (cm H_2O)	0	5	10	15	0
Time started	1200	1215	1230		
MIP (cm H_2O)	34	37	49		
Static pressure	31	32	43		
V_T	700	700	700		
Systolic (respiratory swing) insp.	110	105	98		
exp.	115	110	100		
A-$V_{D_{O_2}}$ (ml O_2/100 ml blood)	4.5	4.7			
Pa_{O_2} ($FI_{O_2} = 1.0$)	60	70			
Pa_{CO_2}	37	37			

Task 15

What would the team do at this point? _____

_____

Assume that the PEEP study proceeded as indicated in the flow sheet below:

Observations

	PEEP steps				
PEEP (cm H_2O)	0	5	10	15	0
Time started	1200	1215	1230		
MIP (cm H_2O)	34	37	42		
Static pressure	31	32	37		
V_T	700	700	700		
Systolic (respiratory swing) insp.	110	105	92		
exp.	115	110	110		
A-$V_{D_{O_2}}$ (ml O_2/100 ml blood)	4.5	4.7			
Pa_{O_2} ($FI_{O_2} = 1.0$)	60	70			
Pa_{CO_2}	37	37			

Task 16

What should the team do at this point? _____

_____

Assume that the PEEP study proceeded as indicated in the flow sheet below:

	PEEP steps				
PEEP (cm H_2O)	0	5	10	15	0
Time started	1200	1215	1230		
MIP (cm H_2O)	34	37	46		
Static pressure	31	32	37		
V_T	700	700	700		
Systolic insp.	110	105	100		
(respiratory swing) exp.	115	110	110		
A-V_{DO_2} (ml O_2/100 ml blood)	4.5	4.7	5.2		
Pa_{O_2} (F_{IO_2} = 1.0)	60	70	63		
Pa_{CO_2}	37	37	34		

Task 17

What should the team do at this point? _____

_____

_____

Assume that the PEEP study proceeded as indicated in the flow sheet below:

	PEEP steps				
PEEP (cm H_2O)	0	5	10	15	0
Time started	1200	1215	1230		
MIP (cm H_2O)	34	37	44		
Static pressure	31	32	33		
V_T	700	700	700		
Systolic insp.	110	105	100		
(respiratory swing) exp.	115	110	110		
A-V_{DO_2} (ml O_2/100 ml blood)	4.5	4.7	5.9		
Pa_{O_2} (F_{IO_2} = 1.0)	60	70	82		
Pa_{CO_2}	37	36	36		

Task 18

What should the team do at this point? _____

_____

_____

Situation 3—cont'd
Observations

Assume that the PEEP study proceeded as indicated in the flow sheet below:

	PEEP steps				
PEEP (cm H_2O)	0	5	10	10	0
Time started	1200	1215	1230	1235	
MIP (cm H_2O)	34	37	52	52	
Static pressure	31	32	34	34	
V_T	700	700	700	620	
Systolic (respiratory swing) insp.	110	105	105	105	
exp.	115	110	110	110	
A-$V_{D_{O_2}}$ (ml O_2/100 ml blood)	4.5	4.7			
Pa_{O_2} (FI_{O_2} = 1.0)	60	70			
Pa_{CO_2}	37	37			

Task 19

What should the team do at this point? _____

_____

_____

Instructor sign off

_____

Situation 3—cont'd

It is now the sixth day of ventilation. V_T is still 700 ml. MIP is 50, and PEEP is still 10 cm H_2O. It has been possible to reduce the FI_{O_2} each day. Today the Pa_{O_2} is 91 with an FI_{O_2} of 0.4.

Task 20

Is it safe to reduce the PEEP?

☐ Yes
☐ No, for the following reasons: _____

_____

Task 21

If you consider it safe to reduce PEEP, write the appropriate orders below:

_____

_____

_____

It is now 1700 hours (5 PM) on the seventh hospital day. The patient is alert, T = 37.8, HR = 100, BP = 120/80. The patient is triggering the ventilator 16 times per minute. V_T = 700 ml. PEEP has been reduced to zero. The peak pressure is now 30 cm H_2O. VC = 825 ml. He can generate inspiratory pressures of -20 to -22 cm H_2O. On 40% oxygen, Pa_{O_2} = 65, Pa_{CO_2} = 40, pH = 7.40

Task 22

Do you believe that this patient is ready for weaning?

Instructor sign off

☐ Yes
☐ No, for the following reasons: _____

_____

Task 23

If you believe the patient is ready for weaning, write the orders for the next step(s): _____

_____

_____

_____

At 0800 (8 AM) the next day, the patient's condition is still satisfactory. Weaning is begun. The patient is given a trial session with the T piece and monitored. After 20 minutes, the patient is returned to the ventilator, which is adjusted to the original settings.

	Still on "assist"	On T-piece				Back on "assist"
Time	0800	0805	0810	0815	0820	0825
f	10	14	15	16	16	10
BP	120/70	120/60	120/70	130/80	125/80	120/80
HR	100	110	110	115	110	105
PVCs	0	0	0	0	0	0
Accessory muscles	0	0	0	0	0	0
Distress	0	0	0	0	0	0
V_T	700	620	580	540	530	700
VC	825				800	
Pa_{O_2} (0.4)	65				60	
Pa_{CO_2}	40				38	
pH	7.40				7.38	

Task 24

Did the patient pass the challenge?

☐ Yes

☐ No, the challenge should have been discontinued at _____ hours.

Task 25

Write your orders for the next step: _____

_____

_____

_____

_____

Ventilator application situation 4

A typical student team consists of an MD, an RN, and an RT. Situation 4 is designed to simulate the problems of a patient with chest trauma resulting in a flail segment.

1. Briefly explain the purpose of the sessions and the exercises.
2. Explain that you will provide simulated blood gas test results whenever the team wants these data but that requests must be submitted in writing on the form that is provided.
3. Distribute Situation 4, tasks 1 to 6, and the blood gas test requisition forms. Instruct the team to check with you after each task. Call attention to this book and explain that all decisions will be arbitrated on the material in the book.
4. Withdraw from the team slightly, and let the team members reach consensus on each decision. When you are consulted, ask the team's reasons for each of its recommendations. Point out those recommendations that are not consistent with the book. (Avoid implications of "right" and "wrong." Instead, point out what is recommended and in accordance with the rationale.)
5. Task 6 requires the team to obtain blood gas test results after the patient has been attached to the ventilator for 20 minutes. Feed back results that are not close enough to the team's stated goals. This will simulate the initial trial-and-error process that is usually required to achieve the desired blood gas levels with a patient-ventilator system. Have the team calculate a new f' and/or V_T' at least twice. Insist that all data be entered in the flow sheet promptly as they are obtained.
6. When the team has completed tasks 1 to 6, distribute tasks 7 and 8, which are concerned with determining the patient's readiness for weaning. The team is required to decide in late afternoon whether to try the T piece the next morning or to wait until the patient is in better shape. The decision should be arbitrated by referring to the appropriate chapter of the book. In these tasks, the team is not required to simulate any adjustments on the ventilator.
7. When the team has completed tasks 7 and 8, distribute tasks 9 and 10, in which the results of a hypothetical 20-minute trial session with the T piece are provided. The team is required to decide whether the patient has "passed" or "failed" the challenge. The team is also required to make recommendations about the next steps in weaning the patient. Tasks 9 and 10 do not require the team to simulate the T piece setup or standby settings.

Situation 4 Your patient is a 30-year-old service station attendant. His chest was crushed today when a car slipped off the grease rack. The patient has a large flail segment on the right. His respiratory rate is 40. His blood gas levels when he is breathing room air are as follows: $Pa_{O_2} = 55$, $Pa_{CO_2} = 30$, pH = 7.48, BE = O, $HCO_3 = 22$. The patient weighs 55 kg.

Task 1

Intubation and mechanical ventilation are indicated because:

☐ Pa_{O_2} cannot be maintained above 50 mm Hg by increasing $F_{I_{O_2}}$.
☐ Pa_{CO_2} has risen above 50 mm Hg and forced pH below 7.25.
☐ Effective ventilation has become inefficient and/or exhausting (f greater than 30 or VC less than 20 ml/kg)

Instructor sign off (Enter time)

☐ Other (specify) _____

_____

Task 2

Specify your treatment goals in terms of Pa_{O_2}, Pa_{CO_2}, and pH:

1. Keep Pa_{O_2} at _____
2. Keep Pa_{CO_2} at _____ and pH at _____

Task 3

Specify the type of ventilator preferred in this case:

☐ Pressure-cycled
☐ Volume-cycled

Task 4

Specify the initial ventilator settings that you would use:

	V_T	f	I : E	Flow rate	$F_{I_{O_2}}$	Sensitivity	Sigh

Task 5

Initiate ventilation in accordance with the above settings. (Use a bag or a bellows to simulate the patient's lungs.) Have your instructor check when you are ready.

Task 6

Assume that you have ventilated the patient at your initial settings for 10 to 20 minutes. Evaluate your settings and adjust as necessary.

Blood gas test results must be obtained from the laboratory.

Requisitions must be marked with the time of the sample and with $F_{I_{O_2}}$ and $\dot{V}_E$ prevailing at that time.

In making your adjustments, you may assume the following relationship between old and new values:

$$V_T \cdot f \cdot Pa_{CO_2} = V_T' \cdot f' \cdot Pa_{CO_2}'$$

Enter all data on the flow sheet below.

When you have achieved your goals, check with your instructor.

Date/hour:	Base-line						
FI_{O_2}							
Pa_{O_2}							
BE/HCO_3							
pH							
Pa_{CO_2}							
$\dot{V}_E$	—						
V_T	—						
f							
I:E ratio	—						
IFR	—						
Control/assist	—						
MIP							
Dynamic compliance	—						
Static pressure	—						
Static compliance	—						

Situation 4— cont'd

It is 1700 hours (5 PM) on the twelfth hospital day. The patient has been doing well. Inflation pressures have been dropping steadily over the last few days. The flail segment seems stable, and chest x-ray film is clear. T = 37.5, HR = 80, BP = 110/75.

The patient is triggering the ventilator at a rate of 12 BPM. V_T = 600. VC is tested and is in excess of 1000 ml when the patient is breathing room air. The patient is able to generate inspiratory pressures in excess of −25 cm H$_2$O. MIP = 18 cm H$_2$O. Pa$_{O_2}$ = 75, Pa$_{CO_2}$ = 41, pH = 7.38.

Task 7

Do you believe that this patient is ready for weaning?

☐ Yes

☐ No (give reason) _____

_____

211

Task 8

If you believe that the patient is ready for weaning, write the orders for the next step(s): _____

_____

_____

_____

_____

At 0800 hours (8 AM) the next day, the patient's condition is still satisfactory, and weaning is begun. He is given a trial session with the T piece with F_{IO_2} maintained at 0.21. He is monitored. After 20 minutes, he is returned to the ventilator, and the original settings are resumed.

Observations

	Still on "assist"	On T-piece				Back on "assist"
Time	0800	0805	0810	0815	0820	0825
f	12	13	13	14	14	
BP	110/75	115/70	115/70	120/75	125/75	115/70
HR	80	85	90	90	95	85
PVCs	0	0	0	0	0	0
Accessory muscles	0	0	0	0	±	0
Distress	0	0	0	0	"tired"	0
V_T	600	550	540	520	500	600
VC	1000				900	
Pa_{O_2} (0.21)	75				71	
Pa_{CO_2}	41				45	
pH	7.38				7.36	

Task 9

Did the patient pass the challenge?

☐ Yes
☐ No, the patient failed at _____ hours.

Task 10

Write your orders for the next step: _____

_____

_____

Ventilator application situation 5

To instructors   A typical student team consists of an MD, an RN, and an RT. Situation 5 is designed to simulate the case of a patient who has ineffective ventilation because of near-drowning.

1. Briefly explain the purpose of the sessions and the exercises.
2. Explain that you will provide simulated blood gas test results whenever the team wants these data but that requests must be submitted in writing on the form that is provided.
3. Distribute Situation 5, tasks 1 to 6, and the blood gas test requisition forms. Instruct the team members to check with you after each task. Call attention to this book, and explain that all decisions will be arbitrated on the material in the book.
4. Withdraw from the team slightly, and let the team members reach consensus on each decision. When you are consulted, ask the team's reasons for each of its recommendations. Point out those recommendations that are not consistent with the book. (Avoid implications of "right" and "wrong." Instead, point out what is recommended and in accordance with the rationale.)
5. Task 6 requires the team to obtain blood gas test results after the patient has been attached to the ventilator for 20 minutes. Feed back results that are not close enough to the team's stated goals. This will simulate the initial trial-and-error process that is usually required to achieve the desired blood gas levels with a patient-ventilator system. Have the team calculate a new f' and/or V_T' at least twice. Insist that all data be entered in the flow sheet promptly as they are obtained.
6. When the team has completed tasks 1 to 6, distribute tasks 7 and 8, which require the team to make a decision about the desirability of applying PEEP. The team should consult the first page of the PEEP algorithm (p. 119). The team is required to write orders initiating a PEEP study but is not required to simulate any adjustments on the ventilator.
7. When the team has completed tasks 7 and 8, distribute task 9. This exercise requires the team to decide whether the PEEP study should be continued.

Situation 5   Your patient is a 13-year-old boy who was discovered at the bottom of a local swimming hole by his playmates. They applied mouth-to-mouth resuscitation, and the boy resumed breathing within 2 minutes. He recovered consciousness but seemed confused. He was hospitalized 50 minutes after rescue. Blood gas tests showed: $Pa_{O_2} = 67$, $Pa_{CO_2} = 36$, pH = 7.42. T was 27, HR = 95, BP = 100/50, $f = 30$.

He was observed in the ICU 4 hours later. His f had increased to 37, T to 38.7. Because of peripheral cyanosis, he was given 40% O_2 by mask, which resulted in $Pa_{O_2} = 60$, $Pa_{CO_2} = 42$, pH = 7.33. He weighs 65 kg.

Task 1

Intubation and mechanical ventilation are indicated because:

☐ Pa_{O_2} cannot be maintained above 50 mm Hg by increasing $F_{I_{O_2}}$
☐ Pa_{CO_2} has risen above 50 mm Hg and forced pH below 7.25
☐ Effective ventilation has become inefficient and/or exhausting (f greater than 30 or VC less than 20 ml/kg)

☐ Other (specify) _____

_____

Task 2

Specify your treatment goals in terms of Pa_{O_2}, Pa_{CO_2}, and pH:

1. Keep Pa_{O_2} at _____
2. Keep Pa_{CO_2} at _____ and pH at _____

Task 3

Specify the type of ventilator preferred in this case:

☐ Pressure-cycled
☐ Volume-cycled

Task 4

Specify the initial ventilator settings that you would use:

V_T	f	I : E	Flow rate	$F_{I_{O_2}}$	Sensi- tivity	Sigh

Task 5

Initiate ventilation in accordance with the above settings. (Use a bag or a bellows to simulate the patient's lungs.) Have your instructor check when you are ready.

Task 6

Assume that you have ventilated the patient at your initial settings for 10 to 20 minutes. Evaluate your settings and adjust as necessary.

Blood gas test results must be obtained from the laboratory.

Requisitions must be marked with the time of the sample and with $F_{I_{O_2}}$ and $\dot{V}_E$ prevailing at that time.

In making your adjustments, you may assume the following relationship between old and new values:

$$V_T \cdot f \cdot Pa_{CO_2} = V_T{}' \cdot f' \cdot Pa_{CO_2}{}'$$

Enter all data on the flow sheet below.
When you have achieved your goals, check with your instructor.

Date/hour:	Base-line						
$F_{I_{O_2}}$							
Pa_{O_2}							
BE/HCO_3							
pH							
Pa_{CO_2}							
$\dot{V}_E$	—						
V_T	—						
f							
I:E ratio	—						
IFR	—						
Control/assist	—						
MIP	—						
Dynamic compliance	—						
Static pressure	—						
Static compliance	—						

Situation 5—cont'd

Twelve hours after rescue, the patient is delirious. T = 38.5, HR = 110, BP = 110/60. The patient is being ventilated at f = 15, V_T = 975 ml. PAW is 10 mm Hg. With the patient breathing 60% O_2, Pa_{O_2} = 53, Pa_{CO_2} = 37, pH = 7.41.

Task 7

Is PEEP justified at this point?

☐ Yes
☐ No (give reason) _____

_____

Task 8

If PEEP is indicated, write orders initiating PEEP study: _____

_____

_____

_____

_____

A PEEP study is initiated. The following baseline data are obtained:

	PEEP steps				
PEEP (cm H_2O)	0	5	10	15	0
Time started	0100	0115			
MIP (cm H_2O)	38	42			
Static pressure	35	40			
V_T	980	980			
Systolic (respiratory swing) insp.	110	110			
exp.	115	115			
A-$V_{D_{O_2}}$ (ml O_2/100 ml blood)	4.5				
Pa_{O_2} (FI_{O_2} = 1.0)	60				
Pa_{CO_2}	37				

Task 9

Should the PEEP study be continued?

☐ Yes; obtain blood gas studies

☐ No; using 5 cm PEEP has the following unacceptable consequences:

_____

_____

_____

_____

Weaning rounds

Overview We recommend that most patients be weaned at 0800 (8 AM) as the result of a decision made on a daily "weaning round" at 1700 (5 PM) the previous day. This exercise is designed to promote that approach.

Target group The target group is comprised of MDs, RNs, RTs, and PTs who are responsible for patients attached to ventilators. The exercise is aimed at beginners or persons who may not be involved regularly in the care of ventilator patients.

Objectives At the conclusion of this session, the student will:
1. Be able to apply the criteria provided in this book to evaluate a patient's readiness for a "weaning challenge"
2. Indicate a willingness to have rounds, criteria and standard procedures for weaning in his or her own hospital

Time frame Individual morning sessions require 20 to 30 minutes for each student. The afternoon weaning rounds require 40 to 60 minutes for each team.

Setting The individual morning sessions require a table, chairs, and semi-privacy. An office would be ideal. The afternoon sessions should be conducted in a private conference room.

Materials "Weaning rounds—1700 hours"—student version
"Weaning rounds—1700 hours"—instructor version (These follow the student versions.)

Pretest No pretest is required, since learning to make decisions about weaning is included in Exercise 4 ("Ventilator application situations").

Lesson plan 1. In the morning, each student is assigned a 20 to 30 minute appointment with an instructor of the same discipline as the student. The instructor provides each student with the student version of "Weaning Rounds—1700 Hours." (We recommend making copies of each of the student versions for each participant.) The student may request any information he or she wants in preparation for the afternoon team conference ("weaning rounds"). The instructor works from material that includes specific data about each patient but provides these data to students only upon specific request. The student is free to consult his or her book.

2. In the afternoon, the students act as a team, pool their information, and make decisions about each patient's readiness for weaning. If a patient is not ready, plans are made to make him ready. The instructors observe the team and comment.

Post-test No post-test is required. Since the cases are handled sequentially, it is possible for instructors to observe students' increasing skills in information gathering and decision making. Students who are willing to follow the weaning procedure in the book generally move much faster through the problems.

After the exercise is completed, team members may engage in discussions of how to implement "weaning rounds," and protocols for them, at their own hospitals.

Weaning rounds—1700 hours

Background We recommend that most patients be weaned at 0800 hours as the result of a decision made on a daily "weaning round" at 1700 hours the previous day. The following exercise is designed to promote that approach.

Design of the exercise The exercise simulates (1) the actual team rounds at 1700 hours and (2) the individual preparation for those rounds. In this simulation, the team has three patients attached to ventilators.

Individual preparation Imagine that you are now preparing to participate in weaning rounds for your three patients this afternoon. Decide what information you would be expected to contribute to the discussion during these rounds. Gather that information by asking your instructor for specific facts, observations, and measurements about each patient. Feel free to refer to your book.

Team rounds This afternoon, your team and the instructors will meet together. The team will conduct "1700 hours weaning rounds" on the three patients and decide which patients are to be challenged with a T piece trial session at 0800. The team's performance will be judged according to the weaning standards specified in the book.

Weaning rounds I—1700 hours

Patient 1 is a 45-year-old male who, two days ago, underwent a cholecystectomy. Because of obesity and a 30-pack-year history of smoking (no pre-op ABG tests or PFTs), he was left intubated and attached to a ventilator. He initially had significant lower left lobe atelectasis secondary to right main stem intubation.

What information will you want to contribute when the team makes weaning rounds on this patient this afternoon? (Any information you need can be obtained from your instructor. However, no information will be volunteered. Feel free to consult your book.)

Weaning rounds II—1700 hours

Student version Patient 2 is a 63-year-old male with known COPD. He was admitted two days ago with an acute respiratory infection, and acute respiratory failure developed. He was intubated and attached to a Bird Mark VII ventilator. He was treated with antibiotics, IV and aerosol bronchodilators, and steroids.

What information will you want to contribute when the team makes weaning rounds on this patient this afternoon? (Any information you need can be obtained from your instructor. However, no information will be volunteered. Feel free to consult your book.)

Weaning rounds III—1700 hours

Student version Patient 3 is a 24-year-old female "Hell's Angellette" who, while riding a motorcycle with her boyfriend, slammed into a parked truck. She was admitted 4 days ago with rib fractures (fourth through seventh right anterior) resulting in a severe flail segment. She was intubated and attached to an MA-1 ventilator on controlled ventilation with a PEEP of 5 cm H_2O.

What information will you want to contribute when the team makes weaning rounds this afternoon? (Any information you need can be obtained from your instructor. However, no information will be volunteered. Feel free to consult your book.)

Weaning rounds—1700 hours

Instructor version

Background We recommend that most patients be weaned at 0800 as the result of a decision made on a daily "weaning round" at 1700 the previous day. The following exercise is designed to promote that approach.

Design of the exercise This exercise simulates (1) the actual team rounds at 1700 hours and (2) the individual preparation for those rounds. In this simulation, the team has three patients attached to ventilators.

Individual preparation In the morning each team member is given a 30-minute appointment with an instructor. The MD student will meet with instructor who is an MD, the RN student will meet with instructor who is an RN, etc.

At this session, the student will be provided with short descriptions of the cases of three patients attached to ventilators. These descriptions will not include the information (as outlined in the book) that the team will need in order to evaluate the patient's readiness for weaning.

Each member of the team must prepare for weaning rounds by actively seeking the information that is needed—especially the information that the team would expect him or her to provide (for example, the RT would measure VC). These data are available from the instructor's copy of each case. The instructor will provide any data that the student requests—*but only upon specific request.*

Team rounds In the afternoon, the team and instructors meet together. The team is asked to conduct "1700 hours weaning rounds" for the three patients and to decide which patients are to be challenged with a T piece trial session at 0800. The team's performance is judged according to the weaning standards specified in the book.

Weaning rounds I—1700 hours

Instructor version Patient 1 is a 45-year-old male who, two days ago, underwent a cholecystectomy. Because of obesity and a 30-pack-year history of smoking (no pre-op ABG tests or PFTs), he was left intubated and attached to a ventilator. He initially had significant left lower lobe atelectasis secondary to right main stem intubation.

What information will you want to contribute when the team makes weaning rounds on this patient this afternoon? (Any information you need can be obtained from your instructor. However, no information will be volunteered. Feel free to consult your book.)

The following information is provided only on the instructor versions of case problems.

Size 92 kg, 5 ft 9 in

| Ventilator settings | f = patient triggering at 16 BPM |
| | V_T = 950 ml $F_{I_{O_2}}$ = 0.40 |

Ventilometrics

FVC = 1.5   MIP = 18

Inspiratory force = −12 cm H_2O Static pressure = 12

Physical examination

T = 38 R   HR = 92 (Normal sinus rhythm)   BP = 130/80

Alert, anxious; good cough reflex; cough produces minimal amount of clear mucus; breath sounds are generally distant with diminished sounds in left base with rales; bowel sounds are present; requires frequent pain medication (receives Demerol 75 mg. q4h and requests it more often)

Intake and output

NPO; IV fluids for maintenance to cover losses; urine output 30 ml/hr; nasogastric tube drains 200 to 300 ml of bile-colored drainage per day

Blood

Hb = 11.9 gm/100 ml   PCV = 38% K^+ = 3.1   Cl = 92

Pa_{O_2} = 120 Pa_{CO_2} = 35   pH = 7.50   BE = +5

X-ray

Some segmental atelectasis still evident in left lower lobe. Tube above carina

PT status

Receiving percussion and vibration q4h while awake and once during the night; active ROM qid; up in chair and ambulation bid with minimum to moderate assistance; able to do fair segmental chest expansion of left lower lobe

Weaning rounds II—1700 hours

Instructor version

Patient 2 is a 63-year-old male with known COPD. He was admitted two days ago with an acute respiratory infection, and acute respiratory failure developed. He was intubated and attached to a Bird Mark VII ventilator. He was treated with antibiotics, IV and aerosol bronchodilators, and steroids.

What information will you want to contribute when the team makes rounds on this patient this afternoon? (Any information you need can be obtained from your instructor. However, no information will be volunteered. Feel free to consult your book.)

Size

78 kg, 6 ft

Ventilator settings

f = patient triggering at 12 BPM

V_T = 1000 ml $F_{I_{O_2}}$ = 0.35

Ventilometrics

FVC = patient cannot cooperate   MIP = 28

Inspiratory force = −12   Static pressure = 10

Physical examination

T = 38 R   HR = 100 (Normal sinus rhythm, no premature ventricular

BP = 140/85   contractions)

Patient seems slightly lethargic; appears weak and emaciated; inspiratory wheezes throughout both lung fields; copious whitish secretions are often recovered on suctioning; has some abdominal distention; breath sounds are diminished with transient expiratory wheezes; receives Valium 5 mg IV prn

Intake and output

Patient is tube-fed 1500 kcal/day; urine output is "good"

Sputum

Gram stain shows occasional organisms, but no white blood cells (WBC)

Blood

$Hb = 15.2$ $PCV = 50\%$ $K^+ = 3.2$

Blood gas now with F_{IO_2} of 0.35

$Pa_{O_2} = 80$
$Pa_{CO_2} = 34$
$pH = 7.50$
$BE = 4$

Two weeks ago in office ($F_{IO_2} = 0.21$)

$Pa_{O_2} = 60$
$Pa_{CO_2} = 50$
$pH = 7.38$
$BE = 4$

X-ray

Chest x-ray film is clear except for small infiltrate in right middle lobe; infiltrate is described as "clearing" since admission; tube above carina

PT status

Receiving chest PT q4h
Breathing pattern: Too lethargic to cooperate with breathing exercises
Exercise tolerance: Poor (requires moderate assistance with exercises and turning in bed); receiving assistance exercises bid

Weaning rounds III—1700 hours

Instructor version

Patient 3 is a 24-year-old female "Hell's Angellette" who, while riding a motorcycle with her boyfriend, slammed into a parked truck. She was admitted 4 days ago with rib fractures (fourth through seventh right anterior) resulting in a severe flail segment. She was intubated and attached to an MA-1 ventilator on controlled ventilation with 5 cm H_2O of PEEP.

What information will you want to contribute when the team makes weaning rounds this afternoon? (Any information that you need can be obtained from your instructor. However, no information will be volunteered. Feel free to consult your book.)

Size

55 kg

Ventilator settings

f = controlled at 12 $PEEP = +5$ cm H_2O
$V_T = 800$ ml $F_{IO_2} = 0.30$

Ventilometrics

FVC = not tested   Inspiratory force = not tested
$MIP = 32$ $PEEP = +5$ cm H_2O
Static pressure = 22

Physical examination

$T = 37$ R $HR = 82$ (Normal sinus rhythm) $BP = 118/78$

Alert (even when receiving morphine); depressed cough; flail segment "sticky" but not stable; no abdominal distention; scant clear secretions; breath sounds are clear with rales under flail segment; requires morphine sulfate 2 to 4 mg IV q2h prn; "agitated" when medication is withheld

Intake and output   Oral feedings; urine output is "good"

Blood

Hb = 11.0	PCV = 37%	Electrolytes = normal
$Pa_{O_2} = 98$	$Pa_{CO_2} = 40$	pH = 7.41 BE = +1

X-ray   Chest shows patchy infiltrates (slight) over flailing contused area—right upper and middle lobes; tube above carina

PT status   Receiving postural drainage tid (no percussion) for right upper and middle lobes and percussion and postural drainage tid for left lower lobe and lingula; receiving assistive exercises bid

EXERCISE 6

Advanced ventilator and patient management exercise

Overview   This is an exercise written in the form of a case study. Decisions are to be made and discussed as the case unfolds. This case provides an opportunity for an expert in each hospital to discuss situations that are not covered in this book, but that are sometimes encountered in the management of patients attached to ventilators. These discussion areas may be suggested by material in the book, but we encourage the instructor to add other topics as he or she feels appropriate.

Target group   The target group for this exercise is comprised of MDs, RNs, and RTs who are responsible for the management of complex ventilation cases and who have completed the previous exercises in this manual.

Objectives   At the end of this exercise, team members will have discussed in detail the management of a complex mechanical ventilation case. Their discussions will have been based on the guidelines recommended by this manual and also those current in their own institutions.

Time frame   This exercise lasts at least an hour and easily can last as long as four hours.

Setting   Vacant intensive care room or other space that provides the following:
        Space for team members and ventilator
        Chairs
        110-volt AC outlet
        50 PSI oxygen source

Materials
1. Chalk board or flip chart
2. Volume-cycled ventilator
3. Artificial thorax*
4. PEEP device

*This exercise is adapted for the "lung simulator" made for the Manley Lung Ventilator Performance Analyser Co. by Medical Developments Ltd., Beaconsfield, Bucks, England (patent applied for). This device can accept VTs of up to 1000 ml. Two lung simulators operating in parallel can be used to simulate the lungs of patients over 45 kg.

5. Spirometer
6. This book
7. Instructor version of exercise
8. Student version of exercise (one for each learner)

Pretest   No pretest is required. (This unit should follow Exercises 4 and 5.)

Lesson plan   The instructor should be familiar with the case to be studied and prior to the discussion should add to the suggested topics any additional discussion items he or she feels appropriate. The instructor should prepare a ventilator that has a manifold and tubing as well as an artificial thorax.

Post-test   No post-test is required.

Student version

A 45-year-old male is brought to the emergency room following a car accident. He has suffered a severe blow to his chest from the steering wheel of his car. He looks dusky, seems to be in shock, and is minimally responsive. He weights approximately 85 kg. It is 1730 hours (5:30 PM)

1. What actions should be taken as initial therapy after a cursory physical examination?

2. What diagnostic tests should be done immediately?

3. What current and/or potential problems do you anticipate?

The chest x-ray film reveals fractures of ribs 4, 5, 6, 7, and 8 on the right with no mediastinal widening.

After initial stabilization, you decide to transfer the patient to the intensive care unit.

4. What precautions should be taken to ensure safe transport to the ICU?

5. Assuming you have a choice of ventilators, what type would you select for this patient?

The patient is transferred to the ICU while being ventilated with a resuscitation bag at an F_{IO_2} of 1.0 by the nurse. A volume-cycled ventilator is available at the bedside.

Using a test lung, the therapist should now set the ventilator for this patient.

Settings: V_T = _____

                F_{IO_2} = _____

                   f = _____

             IFR = _____

    Sensitivity = _____

6. What other equipment should be available for this patient?

It is now 1815 hours (6:15 PM). The results of the initial blood gas tests on blood drawn in the emergency room have been reported. They are:

    Pa_{O_2} = 42 (face mask oxygen)

  Pa_{CO_2} = 64

      pH = 7.19

  HCO_3 = 23

7. Interpret the acid-base and oxygenation status.

Arterial blood gas levels are determined as soon as the condition of the patient being ventilated has stabilized. They are:

    Pa_{O_2} = 61

  Pa_{CO_2} = 34

      pH = 7.46

  HCO_3 = 24

8. Interpret the blood gas test results. What (if any) changes should be made in the ventilator settings?

The patient is now attached to the volume ventilator, which is operating according to your new settings. You wish to verify the accuracy of your settings with reference devices.

Measure and record:

Maximum inspiratory pressure = _____

Static pressure = _____

V_T = _____

f = _____

$F_{I_{O_2}}$ = _____

Breath sounds are very decreased in the left base.

9. What are possible causes of decreased ventilation in the left base?

10. What actions would you take now?

The chest x-ray film reveals a fluid level at the left base layering out at the seventh rib.

11. What actions will you take now?

A thoracentesis is done. 1000 ml of blood and fluid is removed.

Measure and record:

Maximum inspiratory pressure = _____

Static pressure = _____

V_T = _____

f = _____

$F_{I_{O_2}}$ = _____

Blood gas tests performed after the thoracentesis reveal:

Pa_{O_2} = 85

Pa_{CO_2} = 38

pH = 7.42

HCO_3 = 23

12. Interpret these blood gas test results.

You notice an increase in maximum inspiratory pressure while you are proceeding with the care of the patient. However, there is no change in the static pressure.

13. What action will you take now?

14. What is the result?

   MIP = _____
   SPR = _____
   CMP = _____

Crystalloids are being infused at the rate of 200 ml per hour to maintain acceptable blood pressure, heart rate, and urine output.

Twelve hours later, you notice a gradual rise in maximum and static inspiratory pressures.

15. What are possible reasons for this increase?

16. What action will you take now?

Repeat chest x-ray film shows bilateral diffuse infiltrates.
Arterial blood gases tests show:

$$Pa_{O_2} = 38$$
$$Pa_{CO_2} = 39$$
$$pH = 7.41$$
$$HCO_3 = 24$$

17. Interpret these blood gas test results.

18. What action will you take now?

Six hours later, your patient is being ventilated with PEEP and high tidal volumes. You notice sudden increased restlessness and duskiness and decreased breath sounds on the left. The blood pressure drops; the heart rate speeds, then slows. MIPs are very high.

19. What actions should you take now?

Pre-treatment blood gas tests reveal:

$$Pa_{O_2} = 35$$
$$Pa_{CO_2} = 75$$
$$pH = 7.06$$
$$HCO_3 = 20$$

Needle decompression of a tension pneumothorax is followed by insertion of a chest tube.

20. What actions will you take now?

Measure and record:

Set V_T = _____
Inspired V_T = _____
Exhaled V_T = _____

21. What modifications in therapy are required now?

Gradually over the next weeks, the Pa_{O_2} improves, the air leak seals, the flail segment stabilizes, and your patient is extubated and sent home to take a remedial driving safety program.

Congratulations

PREPARATION BY INSTRUCTOR: Prepare the volume ventilator by placing all settings at minimum or zero levels. Attach the artificial thorax to the ventilator, and engage all three springs on the artificial thorax.

COMMENTS TO INSTRUCTOR: The material in boldface type appears only in the *instructor version*. Read each section of the case study aloud with the students and discuss the items in boldface before proceeding to the next section.

A 45-year-old male is brought to the emergency room following a car accident. He has suffered a severe blow to his chest from the steering wheel of his car. He looks dusky, seems to be in shock, and is minimally responsive. He weighs approximately 85 kg. It is 1730 hours (5:30 PM).

1. What actions should be taken as initial therapy after a cursory physical examination?

    Discuss: **Establishment of airway**
    Need for mechanical ventilation
    Access to a vein and administration of intravenous fluids
    Monitoring that should be initiated

2. What diagnostic tests should be done immediately?

    Discuss: **Chest x-ray**   **EKG**
    ABG tests   **Vital signs**
    CBC   **Arterial line**
    Electrolytes   **CVP line**
    SMA-12   **Cardiac monitoring**

3. What current and/or potential problems do you anticipate?

    Discuss: **Flail chest**   **Cardiac tamponade**
    Hemothorax, pneumothorax   **Atelectasis**
    Pericardial tear   **Shock**
    Internal abdominal injuries   **Arrhythmias**

The chest x-ray film reveals fractures of ribs 4, 5, 6, 7, and 8 on the right with no mediastinal widening.

After initial stabilization, you decide to transfer the patient to the intensive care unit.

4. What precautions should be taken to ensure safe transport to the ICU?

    Discuss: **Resuscitation bag with oxygen supply**
    Portable monitor/defibrillator with constant monitoring
    Constant attention of MD, RN, and RT
    Adequate access to a vein for infusion of emergency drugs

5. Assuming you have a choice of ventilators, what type would you select for this patient?

Criteria for deciding between volume-cycled and pressure-cycled types (The guide to selection of ventilator [p. 15] may be used here.)

The patient is transferred to the ICU while being ventilated with a resuscitation bag at an F_{IO_2} of 1.0 by the nurse. A volume-cycled ventilator is available at the bedside.

Using a test lung, the therapist should now set the ventilator for this patient.

Settings: V_T = _____

F_{IO_2} = _____

f = _____

IFR = _____

Sensitivity = _____

Discuss: **Rationale for these settings (The guide to initial settings [p. 39] may be used here.)**

6. What other equipment should be available for this patient?

Discuss: **Chest tube insertion equipment**
Whole blood, plasma products, intravenous solutions
Resuscitation equipment

It is now 1815 hours (6:15 PM). The results of the initial blood gas tests on blood drawn in the emergency room have been reported. They are:

Pa_{O_2} = 42 (face mask oxygen)

Pa_{CO_2} = 64

pH = 7.19

HCO_3 = 23

7. Interpret the acid-base and oxygenation status.

Discuss: **The mode of ventilation at the time the arterial blood was drawn**
The need for current ABG tests during mechanical ventilation

Arterial blood gas levels are determined as soon as the condition of the patient being ventilated has stabilized. They are:

Pa_{O_2} = 61

Pa_{CO_2} = 34

pH = 7.46

HCO_3 = 24

8. Interpret the blood gas test results. What (if any) changes should be in the ventilator settings?

Discuss: **The fact that mild alkalosis may permit easier control over ventilation**
The fact that, depending on the F_{IO_2} that the student selected, PEEP may be considered
Possible causes of hypoxemia

The patient is now attached to the volume-cycled ventilator, which is operating according to your new settings. You wish to verify the accuracy of your settings with reference devices.

Measure and record:

Maximum inspiratory pressure = _____

Static pressure = _____

V_T = _____

f = _____

$F_{I_{O_2}}$ = _____

Breath sounds are very decreased in the left base.

9. What are possible causes of decreased ventilation in the left base?

Discuss: **Possibility of intubation of right main stem or other tube misplacement**

Possibility of hemothorax or pneumothorax

Possibility of occlusion from injury, foreign body, blood, teeth, etc.

Possibility of splinting, muscle spasm

10. What actions would you take now?

Discuss: **Stat chest x-ray**

Stat arterial blood gas tests

Checking patient-ventilator system for leaks, proper function

Determining need for pain medication

The chest x-ray film reveals a fluid level at the left base layering out at the seventh rib.

11. What actions will you take now?

Discuss: **Thoracentesis**

Chest tube

A thoracentesis is done. 1000 ml of blood and fluid is removed.

Remove the third spring from the artificial thorax.

Measure and record:

Maximum inspiratory pressure = _____

Static pressure = _____

V_T = _____

f = _____

$F_{I_{O_2}}$ = _____

Blood gas tests performed after the thoracentesis reveal:

Pa_{O_2} = 85

Pa_{CO_2} = 38

pH = 7.42

HCO_3 = 23

12. Interpret these blood gas test results.

> **Leave two springs on.**
> **Add a resistance of 50 (to simulate airway obstruction).**

You notice an increase in maximum inspiratory pressure while you are proceeding with the care of the patient. However, there is no change in the static pressure.

13. What action will you take now?

> **Discuss:**   **Airway resistance causing MIP to rise without corresponding rise in static pressure**
>   **Evaluation of need for suctioning**
>   **Looking for kinked tubings**
>
> **Remove the R of 50 after students understand the cause of change in airway pressure.**
> **See the book for explanation and diagrams of the relationships between static pressure and maximum inspiratory pressure.**

14. What is the result?

$$MIP = \underline{\hspace{3cm}}$$
$$SPR = \underline{\hspace{3cm}}$$
$$CMP = \underline{\hspace{3cm}}$$

Crystalloids are being infused at the rate of 200 ml per hour to maintain acceptable blood pressure, heart rate, and urine output.

> **Discuss:**   **Recognition of hypovolemia as manifested by "respiratory swing" in blood pressure**
>   **Need for daily or twice-daily weighings of patients with contused chests, since lungs can accumulate water**
>
> **Add the third spring.**

Twelve hours later you notice a gradual rise in maximum and static inspiratory pressures.

15. What are possible reasons for this increase?

> **Discuss:**   **Possibility of increased lung water with large volume of infused crystalloid**
>   **Alveolar collapse caused by absorption atelectasis if the F_{IO_2} is high**
>   **Pneumonia**

16. What action will you take now?

> **Discuss:**   **Need to reevaluate chest x-ray film or obtain current one**
>   **Need to reevaluate or obtain current weight**
>   **Evaluation of fluid balance and need for diuresis**

Repeat chest x-ray film shows bilateral diffuse infiltrates.
Arterial blood gas tests show:

$Pa_{O_2} = 38$
$Pa_{CO_2} = 39$
$pH = 7.41$
$HCO_3 = 24$

17. Interpret these blood gas test results.

18. What action will you take now?

>**Discuss:** **Need for diuresis**
>**Possible need for pulmonary artery line**
>**Need to increase Pa_{O_2} by increasing V_T, adding PEEP, or both**
>**Note: In this artificial situation, the best "results" are obtained by adding PEEP, since increasing V_T will cause the MIP to rise greatly.**
>
>**The algorithm for determining whether to use PEEP (p. 119) should be followed here. Note: The students should be led to use the algorithm to decide whether to use PEEP.**

Six hours later:

>**Manually hold thorax bellows to produce MIPs of 80.**

Your patient is now being ventilated with PEEP and high tidal volumes. You notice sudden increased restlessness and duskiness and decreased breath sounds on the left. The blood pressure drops; the heart rate speeds, then slows. MIPs are very high.

19. What actions should you take now?

>**Discuss:** **Strong possibility of tension pneumothorax**
>**Need for stat blood gas tests and chest x-ray**
>**Need for needle or chest tube decompression *stat* if circulation is greatly compromised**

Pre-treatment blood gas tests reveal:

$Pa_{O_2} = 35$
$Pa_{CO_2} = 75$
$pH = 7.06$
$HCO_3 = 20$

Needle decompression of a tension pneumothorax is followed by insertion of a chest tube.

Discuss: Importance of having chest tube insertion equipment available for all patients being mechanically ventilated

20. What actions will you take now?

    Discuss: Importance of reevaluating adequacy of ventilation now that a portion of the tidal volume is being lost through the chest tube
    Need for therapist to measure V_T inspired and exhaled during routine checks

Measure and record:
       Set V_T = _____
   Inspired V_T = _____
   Exhaled V_T = _____

21. What modifications in therapy are required now?

    Discuss: Importance of maintaining a patent chest tube
    The fact that one patent chest tube does not prevent a tension pneumothorax from developing elsewhere in the chest
    The need to monitor MIPs and SPRs carefully
    The need to reevaluate the level of PEEP
    The possibility that V_Ts may need to be altered to compensate for leakage through the chest tube

Gradually over the next weeks, the Pa_{O_2} improves, the air leak seals, the flail segment stabilizes, and your patient is extubated and sent home to take a remedial driving safety program.

Congratulations

Glossary

Abbreviations

Abbreviations used throughout this book are identified.

A-a gradient	Alveolar-arterial oxygen tension gradient
ABG	Arterial blood gases
ARDS	Adult respiratory distress syndrome
BE	Base excess
BPM	Breaths per minute
Ca_{O_2}	Content of O_2 in the arterial blood
C_{eff}	Effective compliance (also known as static compliance)
Cm H_2O	Centimeter of water
CO	Cardiac output
COPD	Chronic obstructive pulmonary disease
CPAP	Continuous positive airway pressure
CPPB	Continuous positive pressure breathing
CPT	Sometimes used as an abbreviation for chest physical therapy
$C\bar{v}_{O_2}$	Content of O_2 in mixed venous blood
CMP	Compliance
CVP	Central venous pressure
f	Frequency (ventilatory cycles per minute)
$F_{I_{O_2}}$	Fractional concentration of inspired O_2
FVC	Forced vital capacity
IDV	Intermittent demand ventilation
I:E ratio	Inspiratory/expiratory ratio
IFR	Inspiratory flow rate
IMV	Intermittent mandatory ventilation

IPPB	Intermittent positive pressure breathing
JROM	Joint range of motion
LMS	Left main stem bronchus
LPM	Liters per minute
MAP	Mean arterial pressure
MIP	Maximum inspiratory pressure
NSR	Normal sinus rhythm
N/G tube	Nasogastric tube
Pa$_{CO_2}$	Partial pressure of CO_2 in arterial blood
P$_{AO_2}$	Partial pressure of O_2 in alveolar blood
Pa$_{O_2}$	Partial pressure of O_2 in arterial blood
PAP	Pulmonary artery pressure
PAW	Pulmonary artery wedge pressure
PCV	Packed cell volume
PEEP	Positive end-expiratory pressure
pH	Measurement of free hydrogen ion concentration in the blood expressed as the negative logarithm of the hydrogen ion concentration
P, PD, V	Percussion, postural drainage, vibration
PFTs	Pulmonary function tests
PSI	Pounds of pressure per square inch
PVC	Premature ventricular contraction
P$\bar{v}_{O_2}$	Partial pressure of O_2 in mixed venous blood
RMS	Right main stem bronchus
SIP	Sometimes used as an abbreviation for static pressure
SPR	Static pressure
TORR	A unit of pressure equal to 1/760 of normal atmospheric pressure and expressed in mm Hg
T piece	A device that delivers gas to an artificial airway while permitting spontaneous breathing
V$_A$	Alveolar ventilation
VC	Vital capacity
V$_D$	Dead space volume
V$_{D_{added}}$	Added mechanical dead space
V$_{D_{alv}}$	Alveolar dead space volume

$V_{D_{anat}}$	Anatomic dead space volume
$V_{D_{mech}}$	Mechanical dead space volume
$V_{D_{phys}}$	Physiologic dead space volume
$\dot{V}_E$	Minute ventilation
V_{sigh}	The volume of a periodic deep breath or hyperinflation
V_T	Tidal volume

Terms

Words, phrases, or formulas used throughout this book are defined and discussed.

acidosis A state in which the pH is below the normal range

aerosol A fine suspension of liquid or solid particles in an atmosphere of gas

airway pressure The pressure in the upper airway, usually noted on a gauge on the ventilator

alkalosis A state in which the pH is above the normal range

alveolar-arterial gradient The difference in partial pressure (expressed in mm Hg) between alveolar gas ($P_{A_{O_2}}$) and pulmonary capillary blood gas (Pa_{O_2}) as the latter leaves the alveolus; the rule-of-thumb normal is 30 mm Hg; the formula is:

$$\text{A-a gradient} = P_{A_{O_2}} - Pa_{O_2}$$

where $P_{A_{O_2}}$ is:

$$[(P_B - P_{H_2O}) F_{I_{O_2}}] - Pa_{CO_2}$$

alveolar ventilation Tidal volume minus dead space (resulting in alveolar volume) multiplied by f; this formula holds true if one assumes normal lungs and airways as well as uniform ventilation and perfusion; the formula is:

$$\dot{V}_A = (V_T - V_D) \cdot f$$

apnea control A setting, found on some pressure ventilators, that controls respiratory rate by controlling expiratory time

arterial-venous oxygen difference (A-V$_{D_{O_2}}$) The difference in oxygen content between arterial and mixed venous (pulmonary artery) blood samples; the normal range is 4 to 6 ml of oxygen per 100 ml of blood; it is calculated with the following formula:

$$Ca_{O_2} - Cv_{O_2} = \text{A-V}_{D_{O_2}}$$

arterial blood gas tests A panel of tests resulting in measured values for pH, Pa_{CO_2}, and Pa_{O_2} and calculated values for O_2 saturation, HCO_3, and base excess

assistor A ventilator designed to respond to the patient's inspiratory effort only

assistor/ controller A ventilator designed to function as an assistor or as a controller; this type of ventilator may, in default of the patient's inspiratory effort, automatically function as a controller

bradypnea Unusually slow respiratory rate

cardiac output	The amount of blood pumped by the heart per minute (stroke volume times heart rate)
central venous pressure	The blood pressure measurement reflective of right heart filling pressure
chest physical therapy	Any maneuver, such as percussion, vibration, postural drainage, or breathing exercises, used to move secretions
compliance	Forces resisting expansion of the lung; the reciprocal (opposite) of elastance; expressed in liters per cm H_2O or $\Delta V/\Delta P$
compliance, dynamic	Compliance of the lungs measured during flow
compliance, static	Compliance of the lungs and thorax measured at zero flow (also known as effective compliance)
continuous positive airway pressure	Usually refers to the application of PEEP during spontaneous breathing; some ventilators are designed to permit the application of CPAP through the ventilator circuit
controlled ventilation	Inflation of the patient's lungs independent of the patient's inspiratory effort; can be accomplished with a ventilator or a resusciation bag
controller	A ventilator designed to provide inflation of the patient's lungs independent of the patient's inspiratory efforts.
dead space	The volume of those passages, in the airways of both the patient and the ventilator, in which inspired gas does not participate in alveolar-capillary gas exchange; broken down into:
	Anatomic dead space ($V_{D_{anat}}$): The volume of all non–gas-exchanging passages in the patient, from the upper airway down to the respiratory bronchioles
	Alveolar dead space ($V_{D_{alv}}$): The volume of gas that enters alveoli that have no blood flow
	Mechanical dead space ($V_{D_{mech}}$): The volume of gas between the patient's airway and either the exhalation port or the Y exhalation tubing
	Added dead space: ($V_{D_{added}}$): The volume of the tubing added between the patient's airway and the ventilator tubing
	Physiologic dead space ($V_{D_{phys}}$): The sum of all the dead spaces
elastance	The ability of a substance to return to its resting state; expressed in cm of H_2O/liter or $\Delta P/\Delta V$
end-expiratory pressure	The pressure remaining in the lungs at resting expiratory level
expiratory retard	An uncalibrated adjustment on some ventilators that provides a resistance to exhalation, thus maintaining a higher positive pressure on the terminal airways; not recommended for therapeutic use because of its tendency to decrease venous return and cardiac output; also called "respiratory resistance"
expiratory time	The interval of time from the end of one inspiratory flow to the beginning of the next inspiratory flow

forced vital capacity	The volume of gas measured at the end of forced exhalation after maximal inspiration
frequency	Respiratory rate; the number of breaths per minute
humidifier	A device designed to deliver the maximum amount of water possible without producing particulate water
hypercarbia	Pa_{CO_2} above normal range
hyperchloremia	Serum chloride level above normal range; normal chloride is 100 to 106 mEq/L
hyperkalemia	Serum potassium level above normal range; normal potassium is 3.5 to 5.0 mEq/L
hypernatremia	Serum sodium level above normal range; normal sodium is 135 to 145 mEq/L
hyperventilation	A pattern of breathing that results in a Pa_{CO_2} below normal
hypocarbia	Pa_{CO_2} below normal
hypochloremia	Serum chloride level below normal range
hypokalemia	Serum potassium level below normal range
hyponatremia	Serum sodium level below normal range
hypoventilation	A pattern of breathing resulting in a Pa_{CO_2} above normal range
hypoxemia	Pa_{O_2} below that expected at a given F_{IO_2}
hypoxia	An inadequate supply of oxygen at the tissue level
inflation hold	A pause at maximum inspiration provided by some ventilators; this control is used when measurement of static pressure is indicated and ordered; not recommended for therapeutic use, since it tends to decrease venous return and cardiac output
inspiratory/expiratory ratio	The ratio of the time spent in inspiration to the time spent in exhalation
inspiratory flow rate	The speed with which the tidal volume is delivered by the ventilator; usually expressed in LPM
inspiratory force	The amount of negative pressure a patient can generate with inspiratory effort; used as an indicator for weaning and extubation
inspiratory time	The interval from the start to the end of inspiratory flow
inspiratory triggering pressure	The negative airway pressure that must be generated by the patient to initiate the ventilatory inspiratory phase; also known as "sensitivity"
intermittent demand ventilation	Spontaneous breathing augmented by positive pressure volume delivery in phase with the spontaneous breathing pattern of the patient
intermittent mandatory ventilation	Spontaneous breathing augmented intermittently by positive pressure volume delivery at mandatory intervals, not necessarily in phase with the spontaneous breathing pattern of the patient
maximum inspiratory pressure	The highest pressure reached at the end of inspiration; the rule-of-thumb normal is 2 to 3 cm H_2O per 100 ml of V_T
minute volume	The volume of gas exhaled per minute

oxygen content	The amount of oxygen actually carried in the blood; arterial oxygen content (Ca_{O_2}) can be calculated with the following formula:

$$Ca_{O_2} = (Hb \times 1.39 \times \text{arterial saturation}) + (Pa_{O_2} \times 0.003)$$

Venous oxygen content (Cv_{O_2}) can be calculated with the following formula:

$$Cv_{O_2} = (Hb \times 1.39 \times \text{venous saturation}) + (P\bar{v}_{O_2} \times 0.003)$$

oxygen toxicity	Systemic abnormalities caused by Pa_{O_2}s greater than 350 mm Hg for 48 hours or pulmonary dysfunction resulting from F_{IO_2}s exceeding 0.5 to 0.6 for longer than 24 hours
orthopnea	Difficulty in breathing while lying flat
oxygen saturation	The amount of oxygen actually carried by the hemoglobin in proportion to the amount of oxygen that could be carried by the hemoglobin
pop-off	An adjustable valve that allows a "safe" high pressure limit to be set; when the ventilator generates pressures in excess of this limit, the valve activates and vents the excess pressure (and volume) to the atmosphere; many ventilators have an alarm that activates along with this valve; also known as inspiratory pressure relief valve, maximum pressure release valve, and pressure release valve
positive end-expiratory pressure	A state existing when airway and intrathoracic pressure are not allowed to return to atmospheric at the end of expiration
pulmonary artery wedge pressure	Pressure that is equal to the pulmonary venous pressure and that usually represents left heart filling pressure
shunt	The passage of blood from the right heart to the left heart without undergoing gas exchange, caused by, for example, a lung unit that is totally unventilated
sigh	An intermittent deep breath taken 10 to 12 times per hour that occurs during normal breathing or can be provided during mechanical ventilation
spirometer	A device used to measure breathing capacities of the lungs
spirometry	The measurement of breathing capacities of the lung
splinting	A reflex tightening of the thoracic musculature to avoid chest wall movement that may cause pain
static pressure	A term used to designate airway pressure at zero flow
tachypnea	Unusually rapid respiratory rate
tension	An alternate term used to express the partial pressures of gases
terminal flow	An adjustment on some ventilators that supplies a separate gas flow to the patient circuit to compensate for leaks
tidal volume	The volume of gas exhaled in one normal breath
T piece	A device that delivers gas to an artificial airway while permitting spontaneous breathing

triggering The generation of effort (negative inspiratory pressure) by the patient to initiate a breath

vital capacity See forced vital capacity

ventilator A device that can be connected to a patient's airway and that functions automatically to augment or provide ventilation for a patient

APPENDIX

Ventilation patterns

Introduction Throughout this book, we refer to various ventilatory patterns and adjuncts to ventilatory patterns that can be established with patient-ventilator systems. This appendix will provide schematic drawings and a description of these patterns and adjuncts to help you visualize the airway pressures that result from their use.

Spontaneous breathing The first drawing depicts spontaneous breathing. Inspiratory pressure is represented by the portion of the waveform below the baseline pressure of zero. This negative intra-airway (and intrapleural) pressure is created by the patient's inspiratory effort, which causes air to move into the airway and hence into the lungs. Expiratory pressure is represented by the portion of the waveform above the baseline, which illustrates the small positive pressure that exists in the airway during exhalation. After exhalation is complete, the waveform returns to zero.*

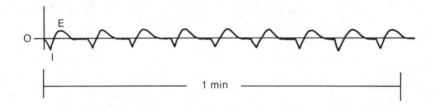

Assisted ventilation Next, assisted ventilation through the use of a mechanical ventilator is illustrated. Just as in spontaneous breathing, inspiration during mechanical ventilation is initiated when the patient creates a small negative intra-airway pressure, which causes the ventilator to "turn on" and deliver the volume you have preset. Therefore, the inspiratory portion of the waveform is represented by both the negative deflection and the positive deflection as the ventilator inflates the lung to maximum inspiratory pressure. The level of this maximum inspiratory pressure depends on the tidal volume you have set as well as on the states of the patient's airway and alveoli. Expiration be-

*In each pattern shown, the vertical indicates airway pressure (cm H$_2$O), and the horizontal indicates a duration of 1 minute.

gins as the positive deflection starts to drop and ceases when the waveform returns to zero.

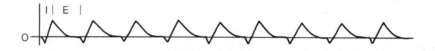

Controlled ventilation

Controlled ventilation is illustrated next. The patient is not permitted to (or cannot) initiate inspiratory efforts. Hence, the ventilator initiates and delivers a tidal volume at a frequency you have preset. During inspiration, the waveform moves from its resting level of zero to the maximum inspiratory pressure. At the end of exhalation, the waveform returns to zero.

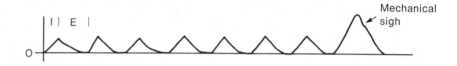

Assist/control ventilation

In the assist/control mode, the ventilator is adjusted so the patient can initiate breaths easily, but if he does not, the ventilator will automatically turn on and deliver a breath determined by the respiratory setting. The breaths initiated by the patient look like those produced during assisted ventilation, and the breaths initiated by the ventilator look like those produced during controlled ventilation.

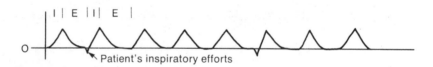

PEEP with controlled ventilation

When PEEP is applied, the airway and lung pressures do not return to zero during exhalation. The waveform looks the same as during controlled ventilation except it is elevated from the baseline by whatever level of PEEP has been applied.

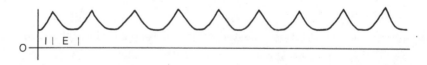

Inflation hold with controlled ventilation

Some ventilators have a control which permits "holding" the tidal volume in the lungs for a preset length of time after inspiration. After maximum inspiratory pressure is reached (at the end of inspiration), the pressure begins falling. It falls until the pressure that was created by airway resistance is released. The breath is then held in the lung for the preset period of time. The level of pressure at which this breath is held depends upon the compliance of the lung and is used to estimate lung compliance. This control is usually used only to measure compliance and should *not* otherwise be used without a physician's order.

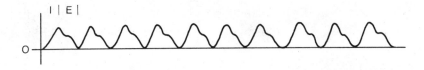

Inflation hold with PEEP   The waveform for inflation hold with PEEP looks exactly like the one described immediately preceding except that the entire waveform is "elevated" above the zero baseline by whatever level of PEEP has been applied.

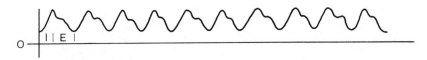

Intermittent mandatory ventilation (IMV)   Intermittent mandatory ventilation is a pattern of breathing that permits the patient to initiate most of the breaths but also guarantees a certain number of ventilator-delivered, preset, volume breaths. The breaths initiated by the patient look just like breaths produced by spontaneous ventilation, and the breaths delivered by the ventilator look like breaths produced by controlled ventilation.

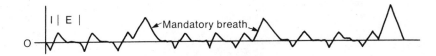

IMV with PEEP   The waveforms for IMV with PEEP look just like the ones described immediately preceding except that they are elevated above the baseline by whatever level of PEEP has been applied.

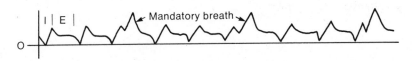

Intermittent demand ventilation   Some ventilators are designed to deliver the intermittent preset volume breaths in synchrony with the patient's inspiratory efforts. Therefore, the breaths that are larger because the ventilator turns on and delivers a preset volume are always preceded by a negative intra-airway pressure component. The other waveforms look exactly like those produced by spontaneous breathing.

Continuous positive airway pressure (CPAP) results from using PEEP with spontaneously initiated breaths. Some ventilators are equipped to provide this mode without using other equipment. The waveform will look like the waveform for spontaneous ventilation except it will be elevated above the zero baseline by whatever level of PEEP (CPAP) is applied.

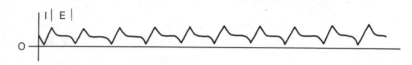